Méric ZONGO

The therapeutic village of ZE KANE Samuel

Méric ZONGO

The therapeutic village of ZE KANE Samuel

bone fracture care practices at Nièté

ScienciaScripts

Contents

A

Defunte MBO ZAMBO PAULINE,
MEYE JEAN MARTIN,
ZE OKOTO Epse MEYE EMILIENNE.

ACKNOWLEDGEMENTS

I would like to express my gratitude to all those who have contributed in any way to the production of this work, and I hope that they will find in these few lines my deepest gratitude.

I am thinking in particular of my Research Supervisor: *Dr Marceline MBETOUMOU.* It was a great honour for you to accept us as students. Your methodological rigour, your sense of a job well done, your advice and your moral and material support are all memorable aspects. You have made countless efforts to ensure the success of this Master's thesis.

To the Vice-Rector in charge of internal and external audit at the University of Ngaoundere, *Pr. BIWOLE FOUDA Jean,* for his financial and material support for this work.

To all my teachers in the Sociology/Anthropology Department, during my academic career.

To all the people of the village of Nko'olong who have accepted me as their grandson, who have worked together to make this study a reality,

I'm thinking of *ZE KANE Samuel* and his son *MONAYONG Martin,* both traditional practitioners in Nko'olong.

To all the patients of the "therapeutic village" of ZE KANE and its enquiries.

To all the administrative and traditional authorities of the NIETE district for their various research authorisations and supervision.

To all my classmates for the mutual help and friendliness that prevailed during the realisation of this work.

To my great sister *MIMBE Michelle Nathalie* for her moral and financial support throughout her years of study.

To my older brother *NZAMBI GEORGES Donald* for his encouragement, advice and material support in producing this work.

To all those who have supported me from near or far with their advice and encouragement and whose names do not appear in this work, not by omission, may they find in these words my profound gratitude.

SUMMARY

The aim of this dissertation, entitled: **ZE Kane Samuel's therapeutic village: bone bill treatment practices in Niete,** is to shed light on the treatment of fractures in a traditional context. This research seeks to understand the process of fracture treatment by a traditional therapist, on the one hand, and the patients' motivations for choosing traditional medicine, on the other. The study area is based on a village in the Niete district. The target population of the study was the local population, mainly patients who had received trauma treatment in the therapeutic village of ZE Kane. When people feel ill, they look for ways and means to regain their health. A methodological approach based on empirical-deductive reasoning was developed following a survey of 31 respondents, including 23 patients, 03 sick nurses and 05 elderly people. This approach led to the formulation of three specific hypotheses which were tested in the field using the theory of social representations (Moscovici 1961) through the concept of the 'central core' and the theory of observational cinema through a 'participant camera' filming interactions. As for the methodological framework, the research is based on the following stages: a summary review of the existing literature on the anthropology of health and traditional medicine, and the development of survey tools. Semi-structured interviews and direct and participant observations were used to collect empirical data, taking into account the specificity of the study area, the operationality of the methodological tools, the study population and the analysis procedures. The results and analyses show that: patients find solutions to their health problems, the reasons for consultations differ from one patient to another, analysis of fractures using a medical image radiography click improves fracture care practices. This study could serve as a basis for decisions by the bodies responsible for health.

Key words : therapeutic village, care, fractures, cliche.

GENERAL INTRODUCTION

I.1 BACKGROUND

In our various communities, we have knowledge, skills and know-how that are being lost through lack of conservation and generational transmission, and which are doomed to disappear. This is the case for the practice of fracture care. Although based on ancestral knowledge, traditional medicine has continued to this day among healers, solely through the oral transmission of knowledge and the practice of the medical art. For Africans, the original concept of nature includes the material world, the sociological environment, both living and dead, as well as the metaphysical forces of the universe. This notion (traditional medicine) is fundamental to understanding traditional African medicine, which in all its forms reflects a way of life, a way of thinking or a culture according to the facet of African civilisation. Bringing this medicine back into the limelight by transferring it from the oral stage, where it is currently confined, to the written and visual stage, will help to revalorise the identity of the African man in his very being: his specific personality and his original culture. GANDO, (2006). The World Health Organisation (WHO) refers to traditional medicine as: "the *body of practical knowledge, whether explicable or not, for diagnosing, preventing or eliminating physical, mental and social imbalance, based exclusively on experience and observation handed down from generation to generation or in writing*" (1976). At the international conference in Alma-Alta in the USSR, organised by the WHO from 6 to 12 September 1978, the WHO recognised that traditional medicine constitutes one of the integral components of public health in States. This opened up the need to give traditional medicine a role in national health systems, which was recognised and accepted by the vast majority of African states.

Despite all these measures taken by organisational and guidance structures with regard to public health policies, some African countries are still unable to put in place an appropriate framework for organising and guiding care. This is the case for the treatment of bone diseases in Cameroon, which is why, when I was asked to choose a research topic, I chose to work on traditional medicine, particularly that used to treat patients suffering from fractures (sprains, dislocations, dislocations, fractures, etc.). This theme: ZE KANE Samuel's "therapeutic village": fracture care practices in Niete. Traditional fracture care has an important place alongside biomedicine in Africa, and in our country in particular. They are rooted in the socio-cultural universe and deeply rooted in the habits of our society, and enable victims of these traumas to be treated.

This medicine, which has a role to play alongside biomedicine, should have the necessary guidance and strategic framework for effective promotion and integration into the national health system. The present work on ZE KANE Samuel's "therapeutic village": fracture care practices in Niete is part of a research approach in social and cultural anthropology, or health anthropology, the aim of which is to understand, question and analyse the logics of perceptions, representations and interactions that guide patients towards the endogenous know-how of traditional therapeutic care practices in the care of patients suffering from physical trauma, particularly bone diseases.

I.1.2 THE PROBLEM

Cameroon has been classified as a middle-income country since 2014, with a GDP of US$32.05 billion, corresponding to an annual income of US$1,445 per capita. However, 40% of its population still lives below the poverty line, defined as an annual income of 269,443 FCFA, or 539 US$/adult. Cameroon's Human Development Index (HDI) is low, with the country ranked 153rd out of 188 countries assessed in 2014. The Inequality-Adjusted Human Development Index (IHDI) has risen from 0.330 in 2013 to 0.344 in 2015, reflecting an increase in inequalities in living standards in the country (PNDS: xv). The current epidemiological situation is marked by a predominance of communicable diseases (Covid-19, HIV/AIDS, malaria, tuberculosis, etc.) and a significant increase in non-communicable diseases, in particular cardiovascular diseases, cancers, mental illnesses and road traffic injuries. Typically, research into illness identifies the criteria according to which patients choose a particular care system, depending on the nature of the illness, the 'affordability' or cost of care and medication, the geographical accessibility of care facilities, ethnicity, social status, adherence to the so-called modern or ancient social order, religious beliefs, in short, the orientation of their mental structures and philosophy of life. EDJENGUELE (2009). Similarly, studies of medical pluralism in Africa have tended to focus on criteria relating to the effectiveness and accessibility of available therapeutic remedies, with the idea of the prevalence of the conventional system in the background, as part of an interface between African medicine and biomedicine. It is not uncommon for some of these studies to evoke the complementarity of the two types of medicine, or the desired revolution from traditional medicine to modern medicine, which is seen as the example to follow. Our study focuses on ZE KANE Samuel's 'therapeutic village': fracture care practices in Niete. Despite the many complications observed in traditional fracture care practices, our aim is to find out how traditional healers and their practices manage to treat fractures. This raises questions about the contribution of traditional medicine to fracture care, and about the rationale for directing patients towards a particular health system, particularly in ZE Kane's 'therapeutic village'.

I.1.3. THE PROBLEM

The practice of treating fractures and patients suffering from physical trauma has an important place alongside traditional medicine in our country. They are rooted in the socio-cultural universe and deeply rooted in the habits of our society, and help to relieve the victims of these illnesses and traumas. Despite the prowess of traditherapeutes' patient care practices, they and their practices continue to be stigmatised. There is no real legal framework for the expression of care practices. As a young researcher and ethno-cinematographer, our aim is to find out what happens in terms of care practice, perception, representation and interaction in this therapeutic village, which is distinct from the modern hospital. Using an ethnographic film approach, I will explore who uses the village, how fracture patients are cared for, and attempt to analyse what underpins patients' choice of a therapeutic village in the event of a fracture. To make the issue of fracture care in a therapeutic village more intelligible, I have chosen to tell the story of these care practices through ethnographic documentary film, because the film shows us the patient's care process by using Jean Rouch's 'participant camera' approach, filming and filming in interaction, which enables us to grasp the activities involved in patient care. Similarly, for an in-depth analysis of the issue, I will draw on Moscovici's theory of social representations in an attempt to understand patients' representations of traditional practices in general and fracture care in particular in ZE Kane's therapeutic village. To carry out this research, the question is what tools are needed to describe, analyse and understand fracture care practices in a 'therapeutic village'? In a 'therapeutic village', what are the reasons why patients turn to particular healthcare systems? In the face of these fractures, what are the patient care activities that enable us to describe, analyse and understand the practice of patient care and recourse in a 'therapeutic village', and how do public health policies provide a framework for the legal expression of therapeutic villages? What methods and tools can be used to interpret bone disease care practices? And what are the practices used by traditional therapists that enable us to understand the rationale behind referring patients to "therapeutic villages"? These are just some of the questions we will be seeking to answer in the course of our work.

I.2.1. History of the subject

The story of our research topic begins in the classroom. In March 2020, during our Film Protocol course with Dr Mbetoumou Marceline, lecturer at the FALSH/UN, we were asked to propose a research topic for our Master 2 dissertations. Passionate about artistic movements of the body and the rhythm that accompanies these movements, and remembering the 'Mbaya' initiation dance of the Pygmees of Adjap-Yesssok in the Niete Arrondissement, I proposed a subject that I felt was relevant to the subject: The Mbaya initiation dance among the pygmies of Adjap-Yessok in the Niete district". I had a burning desire to observe, capture, understand and analyse the symbolism of this dance among this people. But, given the irregularity of this prestigious event among this people, I found it difficult to be on the ground during the period that the university administration allows students to carry out their Master's research work. Even if the actors had to be mobilised to carry out the work, as was the case with Jean-Rouch's *'L'mitiation a la danse des possedes'*, there wouldn't be enough time. So I was asked to think about another theme. It's a case of the opportunity making the thief, the health crisis that is awakening all the components of health in the world, be it biomedicine, traditional African medicine, learned medicine (Chinese, Indian, American...) to come to terms with the corona virus pandemic that is sweeping the world. In March 2020, the month when the first cases of this pandemic were reported in Cameroon, all the health professionals in Cameroon began proposing solutions. The call went out to traditional pharmacopoeias, traditional practitioners, naturopaths, phytotherapists and "grandmother's recipes" - in short, any recipe that could limit the spread of the corona virus disease. The WHO had already declared that traditional medicine and biomedicine should work together, as this would give traditional medicine a higher profile. Initiatives in this direction have led to meetings at the highest level of government between members of parliament and promoters of traditional medicine, the tradi-therapists, on 25 June 2020 in a "special plenary session at the National Assembly on traditional medicine, which is an opportunity for the well-being of Cameroonians". The National Assembly has therefore taken up this preoccupation dictated by current events, traditional medicine, its prowess and its assets. Stimulating debate on a field often equated with charlatanism. To shed light on practices, knowledge and skills that non-initiates confuse with witchcraft. Without necessarily being experts in the field, the MPs have realised "the limits of modern medicine in the treatment of Covid-19". It is in this same vein that Azize. Mbohou in Cameroun Tribune N°12123/8322-45e annee du 26/06/2020 (pp 6-7): "*Une synergie pour developpement et la valorisation de la medecine traditionnelle. Seance pleniere speciale a l'Assemblee Nationale a Yaounde du 25 juin 2020"*. Declared:

"Their approach is therefore aimed at building and, above all, mobilising energies to support this promising sector. This is in line with the appeal made by President Paul Biya, who has envisaged efforts and initiatives aimed at developing an endogenous treatment. What's more, the MPs want to improve and enhance the value of traditional medicine, with a view to making it an effective complement to the health services on offer. The people's elected representatives remember that barks, decoctions and other "grandmother's recipes" are a legacy in our societies. For them, it's not a question of rejecting modern medicine, or substituting it, but rather of making them complementary. The Yaounde conference is

therefore an opportunity to publicise the advances and convincing results achieved by traditional medicine. The aim is also to assess the contribution of Cameroonian researchers and local pharmacopoeia.

These initiatives have multiplied, as was the case at the meeting between the Minister of Health, Dr MANAOUDA MALACHIE, and traditional healers held on 15 July 2020 in Yaounde, at the end of which Bishop Samuel KLEDA, Metropolitan Archbishop of Douala and a herbalist, declared that he had treated more than 8,000 patients suffering from Covid-19 using medicinal plants. This health crisis calls into question the monopoly of modern medicine in public health policies around the world, in Africa and particularly in Cameroon, and the sidelining of endogenous knowledge and traditional medical practices. And, because it has been sidelined, I went looking for documentation for work on the issue of traditional medicine. Traditional medicine deals with endemic diseases, pandemics, trauma, and so on. There is a good bibliography on traditional medicine and the illnesses it treats.

But I want to explore the field of bone diseases in traditional care because there is little work in this area. I remembered that in my mother's village, grandfather ZE Kane Samuel is a traditional practitioner who treats patients suffering from physical trauma, particularly bone diseases (sprains, dislocations, dislocations, fractures, etc.) in his 'therapeutic village'. This gave me the opportunity to reorientate my thoughts on the theme: "The "therapeutic village" of ZE KANE Samuel: care practices for bone diseases in Niete". After having formulated the subject, an unfortunate event anticipated my pre-investigation. In fact, before I had submitted my application for selection to Master 2, at the FALSH/UN on 16 October 2020. A month earlier I had been informed that my mother had suffered an accidental fall and had escaped with a trauma to her right thigh. She went to the Adjap-Yessok district medical centre in the village where she received first aid for five days from 14 September to 19 September 2020. As the pain persisted and the foot swelled, she went to Kribi district hospital for a more appropriate diagnosis. The diagnosis revealed a fracture of the thigh (femur) and trauma to the knee, necessitating surgery. The doctors estimated the cost of the operation at six hundred thousand francs (600,000fcfa), excluding medication and hospitalisation. She spent two weeks in the hospital. Given the cost of the operation and the means at her disposal, and after much deliberation, the decision was made to go for traditional treatment at the home of grandfather ZE KANE Samuel. She arrived at ZE KANE Samuel's "therapeutic village" on 03 October 2020. It should be noted here that before all of the above, I had already gone five years without visiting my parents. This unfortunate event gave me the opportunity to go into the field for two reasons: firstly to visit my parents in order to have a clear idea of my mother's health and secondly to meet my informants in relation to my research topic.

I.2.2. Motivations

The motivations behind this research work are both personal and scientific.

I.2.2.1 Personal motivations

Two personal motivations led me to carry out this research work. In fact, ever since I was a child, I have seen grandfather ZE KANE Samuel take care of and treat a good number of patients who have suffered trauma, particularly sprains, dislocations and bone fractures, and the news of my mother's accidental fall and her decision to go for traditional treatment in ZE KANE Samuel's "therapeutic village" in Nko'olong were two major triggers that led me to choose this research topic. Starting with the polemics surrounding traditional bone fracture care in terms of the quality of care applied to patients, practices, care methods and the resulting complications, I had a great desire to go and observe fracture care practices, I wanted to analyse and understand the reasons why patients are directed to 'therapeutic villages' when they suffer a bone fracture, based in particular on the work carried out by grandfather ZE Kane Samuel and his son at Nko'olong in the Niete district. I would therefore like to explore this field of traditional medicine, which deals with the traditional treatment of fractures in the care of patients who are victims of traditional trauma, because there is little work on this area of research in health anthropology.

I.2.2.2. Scientific motivation

In Anthropology, our research aims to understand, question and analyse the logics of perception and representation of traditional medicine that direct patients suffering from bone diseases to "therapeutic villages" and to show how the knowledge of modern medicine is combined with traditional knowledge, in particular the use of the radiographic image in the traditional treatment of a fracture to make the practice of care effective and efficient - the work carried out by grandfather ZE Kane and his son MONAYONG Martin. For this reason, in visual anthropology, we thought it appropriate to make a film on the care practices for bone diseases, in particular bone fractures.

I.3 Operating concepts :

The Therapeutic Village: according to GANDO (2006: 9), it "*is a therapeutic centre with long-term accommodation*". For us, this is a traditional medical institution offering therapeutic care with accommodation facilities for patients and nursing staff for the entire duration of the patient's care. This is the case for the "fracture care *clinic*" or "nda mvou'ou" run by ZE KANE Samuel at Nko'olong in the Niete Arrondissement, which offers therapeutic care to trauma victims from the moment they enter the clinic until they recover. From this perspective, care is a therapeutic act aimed at the health of a person and their body.

Care practices: Gando (2006:5) states that: "*the conceptual foundations of traditional care based on ancestral knowledge, traditional medicine has been perpetuated to this day among healers, solely through the oral transmission of knowledge and the practice of the medical art*". The practice of traditional care is therefore a way of caring for patients from a traditional perspective. For Africans, the original concept of nature includes the material world, the sociological environment, both living and dead, and the metaphysical forces of the universe.

Fractures: The main functions of bone tissue are threefold: a support tissue (it allows standing and locomotion. Production zone for hematopoietic cells (sternum and iliac crest). Maintenance of phosphocalcic balance. A fracture is a break in the continuity of a bone. There may be a fissure, an open fracture or a closed fracture. Fractures have very different characteristics and evolve very differently depending on where they are located on the skeleton (flat bones, long bones, short bones) and where they are located in the bone itself (diaphysis, metaphysis or epiphysis). Wikipedia defines a fracture as a partial or complete break in a bone. In more serious cases, the bone may be broken into several pieces.

II. LITERATURE REVIEW AND FILMOGRAPHY

II. 1 The literature review

A number of articles, books and theses have contributed to this research. For the most part, these are documents that provide scientific guidance and deal with certain aspects of our theme. This documentary research or literature review is an essential method for verifying and collecting data. It also aims to gain access to relevant oral, written and non-written sources.

According to P. N'da (2006), quoted by Tchoumi Tchouli Elisabethe, (2020:8) "*the literature review consists of a review of the writings. A review is a critical assessment of what has been produced in the field of research concerned*".

In his article "Anthropologie de la sante" (Anthropology of health), Olivier de Sardan (2006) presents a study of two major areas of research in the anthropology of health: popular representations and practices on the one hand, and the modern health system on the other. In his view, anthropology studies illness and health from the point of view of concepts and conceptions, the quest for care by populations and the responses provided by various specialist players outside the modern biomedical health system. Olivier de Sardan believes that ethnoscience has made possible the 'indigenous classification' of diseases. However, the data on this subject has most often been gathered from popular specialists, not from ordinary users. As a result, non-specialist practices and common popular representations have been less studied, despite the fact that these practices account for a large proportion of healthcare procedures. It is also these common popular representations that generally serve as the cognitive or theoretical basis for local healers, and provide a better understanding of adapted therapeutic itineraries. The latter should therefore not only be seen from the point of view of 'tradition' or cultural heritage (although this is generally what doctors and the media ask anthropologists to do). But also from the point of view of DIY adaptation, change and modernity. However, Olivier de Sardan stresses that to study the modern healthcare system, the researcher must analyse its internal workings (organisation of care, professional structure) as well as its external workings (relations with patients and users, and the practices they use). This is the domain of American qualitative sociological studies (with an interactionist orientation). This article now enables us to channel our perspectives and fields of research in medical anthropology.

In his article "*la maladie, un objet pour l'anthropologie sociale*". Fainzang (2000) analyses a number of points which today enable medical anthropology to have channels for orienting research in the medical field, and specifies what research in medical anthropology can focus on. Among other things: the birth of medical anthropology. In order to understand the new knowledge constituted by medical anthropology, it is necessary to overcome the equivocation which consists in seeing this discipline as a branch of the medical sciences which would focus its attention on cultural conceptions of evil, with a view to helping health professionals in their task. In this connection, Fainzang draws a clear distinction between 'medical anthropology' (an ambiguous field, since it is not clear whether it is a branch of anthropology or a branch of medicine) and the 'anthropology of illness' (Marc Auge's formulation to highlight the theoretical implications of these two titles and their respective purposes. This article provides anthropological researchers with channels for orienting their research in the medical field. It explains what research in medical anthropology can focus on.

Similarly, in his article *"Anthropologie medicale dans les societes occidentales" (Medical anthropology in Western societies),* Fainzang (1999) links research in medical anthropology to other fields of anthropology without, however, dispensing with the object of anthropology. At its core, the study of medical anthropology in Western societies makes it possible to examine the field of illness and medicine using categories other than those of medicine, in other words, using truly anthropological categories, since the Western medical institution is an object of anthropological study. Anthropological research has established that there is a close link between the representations that individuals form of illness and therapeutic behaviour in reference to a medical logic that is no longer applicable. All of this exists through an individual's perception of illness and the behaviours they adopt. Fainzang's work on this subject is now enabling new researchers in medical anthropology to open up to new questions, problems that were once considered to be the problems of elsewhere. This work has enabled me to study the provision of care in the 'therapeutic' village, to observe the therapeutic care offered by ZE KANE Samuel in his traditional medical institution, and the perceptions and representations made by the patients who use this structure.

In their article, Abondo. Ngono.R. Et All, 2015 " Cartographie des acteurs de la medecine traditionnelle au Cameroun : cas de la region du centre " in Ethnopharmacologie N°55. The work carried out by these researchers is very important in the context of the promotion and enhancement of traditional medicine in Cameroon in general and in the Centre region in particular. The aim was to identify traditional medicine practitioners and map them in the ten departments of the region. The data collected enabled not only the identification of the players but also the identification of an average of five diseases treated by these traditional medicine players. This work also made it possible to determine the factors contributing to the maintenance of traditional medicine in African states, namely: the Alma-Alta conference in 1978, which enshrined the strategy of primary health care, the success of which depends primarily on the participation of the local population.

Indeed, the health of populations is an endogenous process of development, and therefore requires the mobilisation of available skills and knowledge (traditional practitioners). Then there was the declaration of the decade for the development of traditional medicine (2001-2010) by the Heads of State of the African Union; this initiative was supported by the framework for the development and institutionalisation of this medicine in the Regional Strategy for Traditional Medicine, 2002-2005, WHO/AFRO. Finally, the inadequacies of modern medicine, lack of access to essential medicines (WHO) and the low purchasing power of our populations are also thought to be behind the current craze for traditional medicine. However, there is a vast current of opinion in developed countries which, despite the progress and technological sophistication of modern allopathic medicine, is in favour of promoting alternative therapeutic approaches such as traditional medicine. This trend seems to have been inspired by practices in China and India, among others. As a result of this work, it is now possible to clearly identify the traditional practitioners, their ethnic origins, by gender, whether they are indigenous or non-indigenous to the study site, and the different illnesses they treat. This mapping will enable patients to find their way around depending on the ailment they are facing.

In his article "*Ethnomedicine et anthropologie medicale: bilan et perspective*" Walter (1982) admits that ethnomedicine is a branch of medical anthropology. After drawing up a review of the research published in ethnomedicine, the article shows that the discipline has successively occupied several positions according to the theoretical or practical interest which was recognised in it. Over and above the problems of definition that are evoked, and following a theoretical evolution that is retraced, ethnomedicine today sets out to analyse medical knowledge, taking a global approach or studying the ways in which it is produced, transmitted, disseminated and used; the meaning of disease, tackling the etiological aspect, and studying the different discourses produced, in time and space, on the human body, on health and on disease, on birth and on death; therapeutic studies, which describe cures, present the therapeutic sources of a society or reflect on the effectiveness of a therapeutic system; and therapists, who are studied from the angle of their training, their initiation, the doctor/patient relationship and the social function of the therapist. It also looks at approaches to research in medical anthropology. Ethnomedicine is considered as a subdivision of medical anthropology, a typology which divides the field into three main categories: ethnomedicine, epidemiology and public health. A special place has been reserved for ethnomedicine, allowing the Emic/Etic division principle to be applied to medical anthropology.

The "EMIC" approach consists of analysing the semantic field of certain terms in order to highlight the way in which indigenous people themselves think about and understand certain domains. The "ETIC" approach analyses the distribution of cultural categories in space and time. Referring to these principles, FABREGA (1977) distinguishes two lines of research in medical anthropology depending on whether the disease is seen. Either as a cultural category (this is the Emic approach), in which case we speak of 'illness' in English and 'maladie' in French. Or as a biological category (this is the Etic approach), in which case we speak of 'disease' in English and 'affection' in French. The former corresponds to ethnomedicine and the latter to epidemiology and ecology. In my work, WALTER's work enables me to understand how individuals perceive disease by analysing the sense of perception of disease according to whether the disease is perceived by the individual.

In his thesis Traditional Treatment in Orthopaedic Traumatology: Medical Aspect, Loubna BASSI (2007) examines the medical practices of the 'Jebbars' in certain provinces of Morocco. To deal with this 'illegal' medical practice, which jeopardises the health of citizens, he proposes a multi-pronged strategy to improve access to orthopaedic trauma care: improving road infrastructure, increasing the number of health facilities and improving their management, increasing the number of specialists in orthopaedic traumatology to try to fill the gap in this speciality in several of Morocco's provinces, improving hospital reception conditions and reducing waiting times for patients, improving the social security system to cover the care of the entire population, or at least the vast majority of it. While waiting for an alternative to traditional medicine, and to allow time for any improvements and renovations to be made to health facilities in the public, semi-public and private sectors, he proposes adopting solutions such as: training general practitioners in orthopaedic treatment; these general practitioners, with their knowledge, can detect complications, treat orthopaedically and refer patients requiring specialist advice, thereby reducing the burden on specialist centres and improving access to care. Make 'Jebbars' aware of the risks of complications and the legal proceedings that may ensue. From all of the above, it is clear that studies in medical anthropology have been slow to focus on representations, hospital institutions and doctor-patient relations, and that few studies have been carried out on traditional medical practices. Given that research in health anthropology today is interested in the link between the needs of the population and the health and care responses, this is why, as part of this work, we are going to look at the new practices of traditional practitioners in the treatment of bone diseases, in particular the combination of the two medicines.

11.2. Filmography

In a visual approach, it is necessary to watch films that have a link with the research you want to carry out. In this research, several films contributed to the methodological implementation and narrative framework of my film. These included 'BABY BOOM', a reality film broadcast on the Canal + channels. The story takes place between families and a hospital that looks after new couples during the pregnancy and childbirth periods. This film gave me the opportunity to make a technical choice in terms of expressing emotions: the different shots and camera movements allow viewers to experience strong emotions during the woman's labour process.

In his film "Initiation a la danse des possedees" (Initiation to the dance of the possessed), Jean Rouch clearly defines the narrative framework: we can identify the situational shots, a clearly presented introduction, the body of the film presenting the different activities, relevant transitional images that allow the different sequences of the film to be arranged, and a conclusion - all of which help to tell the story of the initiation activities.

So it was through these films that I made the narrative choices in Ekpwele dokita Bi-vese "The incision of the bone doctor" to give an account of fracture care practices in the therapeutic village of ZE Kane.

III. The main question

How patients are cared for in a therapeutic village

III.1. Specific questions.

1) What characterises the socio-professional categories using the ZE Kane therapeutic village?

2) How does the orientation and choice of traditional medicine in the treatment of fractures help to understand patients' recourse to therapeutic villages?

3) How are patients treated or how is care provided for trauma patients in a therapeutic village?

III.2 The main hypothesis

There are economic, social, mystical and symbolic reasons for using this special traditional health structure to repair fractures.

111.3. Specific hypotheses

1. The therapeutic village of ZE Kane is used for economic reasons (the cost of treating a patient varies between 20,000 and 50,000).

2. Social reasons determine the choice of the therapeutic village (free hospitalisation, solidarity between patients, etc.).

3. Mystical reasons lead patients to therapeutic villages (the fracture is not lost as a simple fact of the accident, but rather as a fact provoked by the enemy).

111.4. Main objective

The main aim of this research is to use a filmic approach to capture the process of caring for a patient suffering from bone trauma in a therapeutic village.

III. 4.1. Specific objectives

Specifically, we will :

a) use the images to describe the process of preparing the remedies, making the object of immobilisation, the treatment (massage, scarification, armouring) and the interactions (carer/sufferer, patient/patient, patient/population).

b) Interpreting the activities of objects used by therapists to care for patients in a therapeutic village.

c) Analysing care activities in a therapeutic village in relation to biomedicine Interpreting and understanding the rationale for referring patients to therapeutic villages.

III.5. THE BENEFITS OF RESEARCH

The work we wish to carry out is fundamental research in the field of social and cultural anthropology, specifically in the field of health anthropology. At the end of this work two interests can be determined, namely the scientific interest and the applied interest.

III.5.1. The fundamental interest

This research will provide health anthropology with knowledge about endogenous knowledge, methods and practices for treating bone diseases in particular (fractures, sprains, dislocations, etc.). As Fainzang (2000:11) states:

"Examining problems relating to health and illness from an anthropological perspective can help to enrich medical research".

III.5.2. Practical benefits

Applied interest will enable the bodies responsible for health (WHO, Minsante,) MINAC, UNESCO, to have a tool for decision-making regarding the care of a certain type of disease, particularly bone fractures, the conservation of therapeutic practices and the promotion of endogenous knowledge and know-how.

III.6.1. The study population

In our study, the study population is made up of the nursing staff of the "therapeutic village", the patients, the nursing staff and the men and women of the village who have knowledge of the history of this therapeutic village, as well as the nursing staff of the Adjap District Medical Centre.

III.6.1.2. Filmic aspects

Specifically, the actors in our film will be chosen from among the patients who come to this "therapeutic village" for treatment of fractures and the traditional practitioners.

IV. METHODOLOGY

The methodology of our research consists of presenting the necessary steps that contributed to the acquisition of results for the benefit of our research. To begin with, we will use the methods of classical anthropology, in particular the qualitative method through observations and interviews. From there, we will move on to the method of visual anthropology, which is the use of the audiovisual tool 'the camera'. The camera heralds the production of an ethnographic film and the main purpose of this film is to show with actions what cannot be explained with words, i.e. the non-verbal, or even more, to give the slightest detail of an action that is considered useless and futile.

IV.1. THE HEURISTIC PHASE

In this part, we're going to talk about exploratory research, documentary research. In fact, this phase enabled me to leave my laboratory, where I had thought up the subject, and get in touch with my field, to observe the fact in question as it presented itself in reality. It enabled me to define my subject more clearly and think about my research methodology more carefully. Documentary research and film research. This is any approach or shortcut used to solve a problem in order to produce solutions in a limited time. In this section, we will talk about pre-investigation, documentary research and filmography.

IV.2 Exploratory surveying

Also known as exploratory research, pre-investigation is a vital stage in all scientific research and anthropology is no exception. After putting our research questions in order, we decided to carry out a pre-investigation, a shortcut that allows us to determine how far, how and how long we are going to stay in the field. With the pre-investigation, we guided ourselves on what we needed to do, the type of information we wanted to have and how to get in touch, if possible, with the population concerned. In the visual part, we'll be doing feasibility studies on the nature of the film we're going to produce, i.e. giving us the opportunity to find out more about the tools needed for recording, the different shots, movements and angles to be taken in the film production process, noise, sound and light. Exploring our field of study is also a way of confirming whether the questions we developed at the outset correspond to what is seen in the field, but if this is not the case, the possibility of reformulating our research questions is strongly considered. To be effective, we need to observe carefully, with a great deal of reflexivity about what we think is best to produce.

IV.3. The start of exploration

In our work, it began on 12 November 2020, when I went to ZE KANE Samuel's "therapeutic village". During the two weeks I spent there, I observed ZE KANE's work in the treatment of bone diseases, in particular bone fractures. It was also a question for me of observing the structure which receives the patients, to see to what extent I can negotiate the realization of an ethnographic film on the practice of the care of the diseases of the bones. I left Ngaoundere on Thursday 12 November 2020, where I was staying at 5.15pm, for Yaounde, where I arrived the next day at 10.45am via the tourist travel agency. Immediately at 11.15am I bought my ticket for Kribi from La Kribienne travel agency. It was due to leave at 12 noon, but after a few hassles due to the state of the vehicles and the lack of passengers, and the staff not wanting to refund my money so that I could change transport agencies, it was finally at 4pm that we left Yaounde with a 70-seater bus that was half-full. I should note here that my last trip to this transport agency was in 2015, so I had very good memories of the quality of service provided by this agency, which was the pride of the Kribi-Yaounde line. But in 2020 it remains a shadow of its former self.

On the bus, I met a lady called Sabine, my seatmate, who was going to Kribi for the first time for a short stay. We chatted during the journey and I introduced myself to her as a Visual Anthropology student at the University of Ngaoundere. We talked about what anthropology studies in general, and the purpose of visual anthropology in particular. From her, I discovered that she is an action film personal responsible for the actors' costumes. She shared with me her experience of film sets. Her role is to decorate the set and suggest costumes to the actors for the different sets. Fifty kilometres from Yaounde, we found a bus belonging to La Kribienne agency that had broken down. We picked up some of the passengers who were still there. They told us that they had set off at 9am and that the agency had been unable to send another bus fifty kilometres away. After these passengers had boarded, we arrived at the BOUM-NYEBELL peage where six passengers had disembarked and two others had set off with us. One of these two passengers introduced himself as a "naturopathic biochemist" who said he had studied at the biomedical faculty of the University of Dschang; he was promoting medicines made from bark from the Amazon forest (a product of American learned medicine). The main product he was promoting was "Natural Skin", a product which, according to him, combats fatigue, cell ageing, blood purification, etc. This medicine comes in tablet form and costs 80,000 CFA francs per box. And since he couldn't find any buyers for the box of tablets, he sold 15 tablets at 2000 fcfa. The dosage consisted of taking three tablets for five days, renewable after two years. Several passengers were seduced by the man's speech and bought the medicine.

This man, aged 42, who liked to say it, and whose physique gave him away as being in his thirties, was eloquent and brilliant in his speeches; he knew all about medicinal plants and their scientific names. He knew how to keep the passengers in such a friendly mood that we almost forgot the difficulty of our journey. He also presented another product, "a stone", which he said he had brought back from Rwanda during his many trips. The dosage for this medicine consisted of taking a piece of this stone, putting it in a litre and a half bottle of drinking water, shaking the bottle and leaving it to stand for 24 hours. The stone dissolves in the water and the water changes colour to a yellowish hue, to be consumed in two glasses on an empty stomach for three days to combat (redness, stomach aches, stimulate the nervous system, combat aches and pains...). He demonstrated the stone while telling us stories about women who don't know how to wash themselves and who lose men because they don't know how to take care of their bodies. This gentleman really kept us on our toes during the trip, and all this reassured me of the prowess of traditional medicine and its effectiveness.

IV.4. Meeting with patients and therapists

After a 5-hour drive, we arrived in Kribi at 9pm. In Kribi I was informed of the wake of a cousin from the village who had died a week earlier. I attended the wake on Friday 13 November 2020 from 10pm to 3.30am, the time when I took a motorbike to the village of Nko'olong in Niete, a village located 19 kilometres from the town of Kribi; The motorbike driver asked me for 4500f because of the poor state of the road, but I negotiated and finally paid 3000f. I arrived at Nko'olong on Saturday at 4.45am, where my mum and the other patients were staying. I was greeted by a sick guard who directed me to the dormitory where my mum was, and who was waiting for me.

Photo 1: Bamboo raffia bed

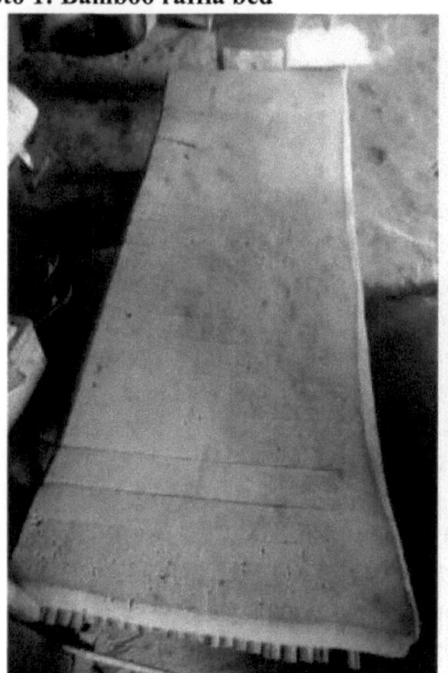
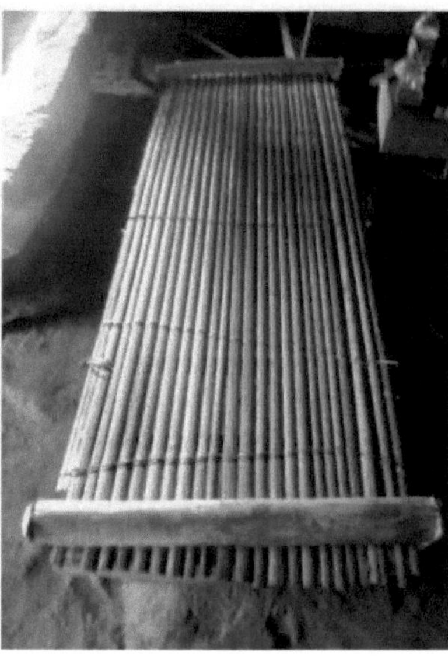

Source: *Photo Meric ZONGO on 18/02/2022 in Nko'olong therapeutic village. The therapist provides his patients with beds and mattresses so that they don't have to sleep on the floor during their treatment.*

Each patient is provided with a bed and mattress throughout their stay in the ZE Kane therapeutic village.

On Saturday morning, 14 November 2020, as soon as I woke up at 6.30am I had this brief conversation with my mum:

QMZ: "Hello Mum

RZE: "Thanks for waking up, how did your trip go?

QMZ: "a very long and painful journey".

RZE: "What bothered you on the way?"

QMZ: "We arrived in Yaounde in the morning at 10am, I bought the ticket at La Kribienne and they told me that we had to leave at 12pm, so I called Michelle to say that I couldn't come over. But it was at 4pm that we set off for Kribi.

RZE: "What was bothering the agency?"

QMZ: "the vehicles were broken down and the lack of passengers, I tried repeatedly to get my money back but they refused".

RZE: "I see, and how did you leave your brother?"

QMZ: "He's doing well, they've got off to a good start with the lessons, and how's your treatment going?

RZE: "It's going a bit, the foot doesn't hurt as much as it used to. My only big problem is that I'm doing everything on the spot.

<u>A heated conversation with mum on 14/11/2020 in the dormitory</u>

She introduced me to the other patients and nurses, where I met three men and five women, allowing me to see six patients and two nurses. The patients included a policeman with a fractured right femur, a pupil with a double fractured left femur, two housewives, one with a fractured right femur and the other with a fractured left, a young girl with a fractured left femur, and a young man with a fractured spine. I go round the beds looking at the patients, each one sitting on his own bed, asking them questions about their state of health while reassuring them that everything will be fine for them and that these things just happen. We're interrupted by a doughnut seller who comes into the dormitory, and the patients make a little bargain, some giving 300f, 200f, 250f, 400f, to buy the doughnuts for the little boy. I left the dormitory to go to the living room to meet grandfather ZE KANE, affectionately called "Papa Moh", who was preparing for the Sabbath because he is a fervent Adventist Christian with whom I had a brief conversation:

Hello "Papa Moh,"

Hello " Petit Moh bonne arrivee

"Thank you.

RZK "when did you arrive?"

QMZ "this morning at 4am".

RZK " How was your trip?

QMZ "a bit well I've noticed that our road is so bad now".

RZK "our trongon has been in this state for a few months now, how did you leave your brother?"

QMZ" he is doing well and so are his studies".

<u>A conversation with grandfather ZE KANE at the salon this Saturday 14/11/2020</u>

IV.5. The start of observations of patient care practices

After this brief conversation I left him to go round the village, saying hello to uncles, aunts, cousins... in short, all the people I knew in the village, everyone wanted to know how I was doing, how I could have spent all this time without going round the village? How are my studies and my health progressing? Everyone had a question that intrigued me: "Where's your wife?" and I replied with a mocking laugh: "She's still in Europe. After this tour of the village, at around 9am, I immediately took the bucket and soap to go and wash at the Ngola river. On my return, the sick warden presented me with the little boy she had reserved for me. It should be noted here that every Saturday, the Sabbath among Adventists, is considered a day of absolute rest, and no activity is accepted by Grandfather ZE KANE, either for himself or for his patients or sick carers. In view of the fatigue caused by the journey and the night before, I went to bed. I woke up at 2pm to find my cousins watching in the lounge. It was around 3.45pm when I heard uncle Aime (MONAYONG Martin), son of grandfather ZE KANE, ask the sick guard to put the pots on the fire. Not knowing what was going on, I rushed to the kitchen to see.

The first thing I noticed was that each patient had a pot under his bed, which the sick attendants took out to heat. In these pots are the barks, the "agnyassa", the black water that the two wardens take turns putting on the fire. Once they had heated up, Carole went to call Uncle Aime. In a friendly atmosphere, the patients listened to music, played Ludo and told each other stories. I'd like to express my surprise at the fact that I didn't know that grandfather ZE KANE had already handed over to his son. I was expecting him to be in charge of treating the patients. When Uncle Aime arrived, he went round the patients' beds, then took a place next to the one he was starting treatment with. That day, he started with the gendarme. He begins by undoing the patient's bandages, removing the 'Akang' made of bamboo and raffia, and the two large pieces of planking used as the traditional plaster cast to immobilise the thigh.

After undoing the bandages, he observes the condition of the place where the shock occurred by tapping. All movements of the patient's foot are assisted by the nurse, particularly in the case of the gendarme. He then began to clean the patient's thigh with the "Agnyassa", which was used as a sponge. He immobilises the thigh with his left hand, while his right hand moves back and forth in the pot of medicine to wet the "Agnyassa" and clean the remedy applied the day before. He repeats this exercise for four or five minutes; once he has cleaned the area thoroughly, he asks the patient for the razor blade and begins to make local cuts (incisions) in the form of sticks. As soon as he has finished, he applies the remedy, a black powder contained in a box called 'Ndoup'.

He repeats the same exercise with all the other patients, who wait in turn. From time to time, the patient who expresses his pain shouts at each other, mocking each other. All of this is done in an atmosphere of good humour between the patients, the doctor and the nurses. After applying the remedy to the patients, he cleans his hands with soap and water and then returns to his activities in the salon. While the remedy is drying, thirty or forty minutes later, he returns to bandage the patients' feet, finishes the bandaging and makes an appointment for the next day at the same time.

I observed this treatment practice for three days before starting to negotiate shooting during the treatment. To begin with, the patients had to adopt me, so I started off by doing odd jobs around the house (cleaning the compound, fetching water, running small errands for patients, etc.), all of which helped everyone to adopt me. I started negotiating with a patient; it was 8pm and we were in the dormitory. As it was hot inside, the patient, who had suffered a spinal injury, asked his mum (who was looking after him) if he wanted to go and get some fresh air in the concession yard. I should note here that of the seven patients, this patient's case is the most serious. He has a fractured spinal column, his two lower limbs are almost paralysed, and he has a catheter to help him evacuate his waste. To get around, two people are carrying him to put him in the wheelchair, and his accident is linked to a fall from the top of a tree. The other six suffered either a left thigh fracture, a right thigh fracture or a double fracture of the left femur.

IV.6. The start of photo shoot negotiations

The nurse and I carry him and I carry his patient and put him in the wheelchair. The patient and I went out into the courtyard, and I took the opportunity to ask for permission to take pictures during his treatment session, which he granted me through this conversation:

QMZ "Dear brother, I would like to ask you something".

RMA "What's the matter, brother? I'm listening "

MZ " By the way, there are two reasons for my trip here. The first is that it's been a long time since I last set foot in this village, and following my mother's accident, I came to see the family and ask about her situation. And the second is that, at school, we were asked to research topics for our Master II dissertations, and the topic I've chosen is grandfather's work, so I'd like, while you're at it, to capture a few images using my telephone, if you'll allow me.

RMA " ah-bon, si c'est pour l'ecole comme tu le dis I ne trouve pas d'inconvenient, et " Papa Moh ", il est au courant ? "

QMZ " Yes, he knows the purpose of my trip, he already knew before I arrived. Thank you very much for your agreement. I'd like to talk to the other patients tomorrow" RMA "OK, tell me, with all the themes you could find in Ngaoundere, what made you choose this theme?"

QMZ "To tell you the truth, I don't know. At first I'd chosen a theme about introducing children to the 'Mbaya' dance among the Pygmies. Then I realised that this event doesn't happen every year and that I needed something to film in order to produce a film, and that's how I came to remember my grandfather's work."

RMA "I see, it's a really good theme".

<u>Conversation with patient RMA in the concession courtyard at 8pm Monday, 16 November 2020</u>

The next morning, after a few small jobs related to cleaning the concession, I had breakfast. After breakfast, Mum and the other patients made a contribution of 3,000 francs and sent me off to buy fish in the neighbouring Nkongtane district. On my return, I gave the fish to Carole, who was responsible for cleaning and cooking. I have to say that among these seven patients, harmony, understanding and mutual aid are the order of the day. As far as nutrition is concerned, they all contribute and the two sick nurses take care of the cooking. From time to time, patients whose healing process is already well advanced are assisted. They are waiting for the final stage, which is the shielding of the treatment. From the kitchen, where I was delivering the fish to the wife of the gendarme who is on sick leave for her husband, I saw a patient under the cocoa tree who seemed to be resting, lying on a mat on the floor. I approached her and told her I wanted to talk to her. She gave me this broken conversation:

QMZ "Auntie, are you getting some air?"

RAL "ah, I'm resting here, it's too hot inside".

QMZ "I can see that your situation is improving (I play the recording on my phone without her noticing)".

RAL "yes, it's getting better, when I had my accident, I decided not to go to hospital, that I would finish my treatment locally."

QMZ " and yes, "

RAL "they wanted me (family members) to go to hospital, but I refused, because I wouldn't do the hospital protocols: come and put the iron on my foot, the cast... ". QMZ "the iron?

I said no, I was going to the village to treat my mvou'ou (fracture). The day I had my accident was the same day I arrived here.

QMZ "wow, and how?"

RAL" is true, I endured the pain and I was on the bike. When I arrived, Tonton Aime first sent me to get an X-ray before I was treated, because he doesn't treat without a click. So I tried to call the people at home so that they could send the car for me, and my little nephew came to take me here to Kribi, where I spent two days. I had the accident on 15 September 2020, and I came back on the 18th, so I'll be here for two months tomorrow.

QMZ "formidable

RAL "It was only a matter of time, God allowed me to walk quickly".

QMZ " really, where I frequent, I have chosen a theme that I would like to do the portrait of grandfather "

RAL "would you like to paint a portrait of grandpa?

QMZ "yes, we've applied to the school but we haven't been accepted yet, we don't know if we'll be attending this year.

RAL "God will help, you just have to pray".

QMZ "if they take us, I think I'll be coming back here in September next year".

RAL "do you support?"

QMZ "no, first of all, let me come and work here".

RAL "I see, you're starting to learn?

QMZ "not to learn, but to understand why people come here for treatment and to film how he massages his patients".

RAL "I understand, I understand and you rewrite your memory".

QMZ "yes, so if we're taken on, we may start school in December 2020, as we're still on holiday".

RAL "I can see why you came back, there's no point in staying there until you've started".

QMZ" yes, we're still on holiday ".

R "It's better to go when school has already started, God will help, you just have to stay in prayer, nothing is impossible to God. So tufinis to write how he massages, how he does it, when he has already finished, he leaves time, then he comes to attach, that's what you're going to support... "

QMZ" yes

RAL "and they ask you questions (teachers)".

QMZ" yes (laughs)

RAL "laughter and interjections "ah yah. oh la, la" that's fine because people like to use the memes, memes memes so we need to change."

QMZ" Yes, because this is where I grew up.

RAL "ah, you grew up here in Nko'olong?"

QMZ" yes

RAL "ok, in your maternal village."

QMZ "yes, when I had... the idea came like that and it happened that mum had an accident".

RAL "yes, I understand, you've decided to do your dissertation on this, you just need to talk to grandpa a lot".

QMZ "yes, he and I are going to have a chat".

RAL "you have to pray a lot God will help".

QMZ "I would like to film with my phone while he is massaging you to get some images of his work".

RAL "no problem, you can film, you can film when he gives us a massage".

QMZ" thank you very much

<u>Conversation with patient RAL on 17 November 2020 at 11.45 a.m. under the cocoa tree</u>

After a few minutes with her, I take my leave of her and meet up with the young girl patient, the young spinal patient and the student with double fractures who were watching in the lounge. I tell them about the social and cultural life of the northern regions and my day-to-day experience of how I quickly integrated into the environment despite the cultural differences. Only the language is still lacking but for the rest I'm trying to adapt. When we broached the subject of school, the first patient to whom I'd been given the go-ahead nodded to me to let me know if I'd already received the go-ahead from the other patients? I immediately took the opportunity to introduce my subject to the two patients who were watching the pupil and the young girl with us and asked them if they would allow me to film their treatment sessions. I then let them know that I already had the agreement of two patients. They both agreed.

The next morning, 18 November 2020, after morning prayers, it's 6.15am when I take the container to the river to make five water turns, fill the basins with water, and as soon as I've finished, I also take the hoe to start weeding the concession yard. It's 11am when I take my break and go and get something to eat. A nurse presents me with my plate of food, which I promptly eat. Two patients are watching in the lounge, two other patients have gone for rehabilitation (walking without a crutch for one and with a crutch for the other), a sick guard is at the river fetching water to drink and another sick guard is cleaning the manioc in the kitchen. There are four of us in the dormitory - Mum, the gendarme, another patient and me. Although I had already established a good relationship with these two patients, and they appreciated me for the services I provided, I had a feeling of fear that drove me to ask to be photographed during their treatment sessions. My fear was explained firstly by the age difference between us and secondly I was afraid of the reaction of these two patients, in particular the refusal of my heartbeat. I watched them for a while, then took a seat next to the gendarme's bed, which was also the bed of the other patient, and let them know I wanted to have a chat with them.

As I did with the other patients, I began by presenting the purpose of my trip, then asked for the images to be taken during the treatment session and why I needed them. I was relieved when the patient said in a sympathetic voice: "my son, if it's for school as you say, I authorise you to take the images, but on condition that they're not broadcast as whatsap". The gendarme also found the subject interesting and asked me to keep the images after making my film and to show them to him. I guarantee them my good faith and that I know how to protect their images. I am relieved once again that they have all given me permission to film their treatment session. I also think that the presence of my mum, who was in the same situation as these patients, played a big part in my decision. Having already obtained the agreement of all the patients, the first filming began at 4.30pm on Wednesday, when I returned from a patients' committee meeting to find grandfather ZE KANE massaging his patients. He had already massaged the two patients; I rushed to the shelf where I had left my telephone in charge. He was now starting with my mum and I immediately looked for a camera angle. I start filming through the window of the dormitory, filming for 12min43s.

He begins by undoing the patient's bandages, the "Akang" and another bandage, observes the evolution of the fracture and then begins to clean the medicine applied the day before using the "Agnyassa" which he puts in the medicine pot from time to time. Once he has cleaned it well, he asks for the blade and then starts to make local cuts in the form of sticks. The patient expresses the pain of the blade by shouting while the others laugh at their cries. The grandfather's great-grandson is playing with a patient, the gendarme and a patient are each sitting on their own bed, a sick nurse is sifting cassava in the kitchen and the other nurse is chatting with her husband, the gendarme. Grandfather ZE KANE explains that, when we massage where the bone has consolidated, it's so that "the lump doesn't come out on that spot and the medicine prevents the blood from clotting", he adds that "when you've had an accident and your chest hurts, you consume this medicine, you consume this powder so that when the blood clots in the chest or in the stomach, this product allows the blood to leave the body". As soon as he finishes applying the medicine to his patients, he takes leave of them and comes back with a bandage 20 to 30 minutes later and the appointment is made for the next day.

The next day I decided to observe the patient care protocol and found that :

All treatment sessions take place in the afternoon. After heating the pots, the traditional practitioner undoes the patient's bandages, then observes the state of the fracture by tattooing, then cleans the remedy applied the day before, makes local scarifications to let the blood flow, and finally applies the remedy. Once the remedy has been applied, the therapist leaves it to dry for 20 to 30 minutes, then returns to bandage the patient's fractures.

I tried to understand why each patient had his own pot and blades for the treatment, and it was the patient Nestor who gave me a few snippets of information on the subject in a casual conversation:

QMZ: "Why do each of you have your own pot and blades?"

RNE: "From what I've learnt, he used to use a pot and a blade for all the patients. But because some patients didn't follow the rules, it slowed down the treatment. When a patient doesn't respect the rules, it shows up in the medicine pot. And so, as was usually the case with patients who didn't respect the prohibitions, he found it better to ask the patients to each buy their own pot and blades. He had one blade that he used for all his patients, and that's when he saw that some patients, when their treatment was finished, could go into the treatment pot and block the treatment of others. It's better that each patient has their own pot, so if you have your spirits, it stays in your pot, so if you have your illness in your blood, the blood doesn't get contaminated through the blade because everyone, everyone has their own pot. Before, there was only one pot for the treatment.

QMZ: "Now you're coming, buying your cooking pot and the necessities he often asks for?

RNE: "yes

QMZ: "So how many blades did you use during your treatment?"

REN: "(silence) well after three or four days you change the blade, after four months here in Nko'olong I can say that I've used four packs of blades. That's often ten blades per pack.

QMZ: "ten blades per pack and the pack costs about how much?"

REN: " 350f"

QMZ: "is it any style of blade or is there a category of blade he prefers?" REN: "well, it's any style of blade, but you're the sick one who prefers the blade, so ga be only one blade, but any blade, any brand, ga be only one blade. Well, it's not based on a brand of blade it's any blade that does the treatment."

We are interrupted by a nurse who asks me to accompany the patient to the lounge.

<u>Conversation with REN on 20/11/2020 in the concession courtyard at 4.15pm</u>

This exploratory research gave me an idea of the constraints involved in making this film. This exploration enabled me to narrow down my subject to the practice of fracture care, to better formulate my problem, and to formulate hypotheses and research questions.

V. Documentary Research

After first investigating our field of research, we will look at the documents or work produced by other authors in relation to our field. According to Magalakwe, who quotes Bailey in "the use of documentary research method in social research" (2006:221): "*the use of documentary methods refers to the analysis of documents that contain information about the phenomenon we wish to study*".

With regard to our problem, we came across numerous documents which made us aware of exactly what we needed to do and redirect our attention so as not to repeat what another author had worked on. In the course of our investigations, we had the privilege, through our documentation, of highlighting the techniques that would be used to collect data, such as the observation and interview techniques we mentioned earlier, as well as the way in which qualitative research is conducted in the social sciences.

In all serious scientific work, good documentary research helps to improve the work of previous authors. According to M. Grawitz, *"the documentary technique consists of a systematic search of everything written in connection with the field of research"*. For the purposes of this work, I turned to works on the anthropology of health, traditional practices, traditional medicine and bone diseases. This documentary research was carried out in several documentation centres, in particular at the Central Library of the University of Ngaoundere, the Library of the Faculty of Arts, Letters and Human Sciences of the University of Ngaoundere, through several Internet research sites, with resource persons and my private documentation. In the light of the various documents I consulted and with resource persons, this documentary research enabled me to better elaborate my problem and my problematic, to better identify the perspective of my problematic on those who preceded me on the question, and to make methodological choices.

VI. THE PRACTICAL PHASE

In this section, we will discuss the location of the production area, the location of the activities, the location of our main stakeholders and the location of the stakeholders to be interviewed on camera.

VII.. Spotting itself

This is done during our immersion in the field of study or production. We want to make it known that we worked in this therapeutic village as a sick guard in order to be adopted by patients and gain their trust with the help and collaboration of therapists ZE Kane Samuel and his son MONAYONG Martin. This approach enabled the patients to feel safe and open enough to help us carry out this research and to know that there is someone who sympathises with their suffering.

VI.2 Locations

The work took place in a traditional health facility offering specialist care for patients suffering from bone fractures. The facilities are the different areas given over to each patient during their stay in the ZE Kane therapeutic village. We also visited the Adjap district medical centre to get a holistic view of the issue of bone fracture care and to contrast the data collected from the ZE Kane therapeutic village.

VI.3. Identification of activities

In our study, which is that of a qualitative approach and being in a filmic approach, our study population is made up of our actors among whom: the choices of these people were deliberately made by their characteristics and their representative to design a non-random sample. All the people included in our study have a link with fracture care or the 'therapeutic village'. In order to determine the size of our sample, we conducted a field study lasting three consecutive months, from November 2021 to January 2022. All cases of fractures treated in the "therapeutic village" of ZE KANE in the Niete Arrondissement.

Our study population included: All the nursing staff of the "therapeutic village", i.e. ZE Kane and his son Monayong, as well as any patient who had received treatment in ZE KANE's "therapeutic village"; People who had been victims of traumatic accidents with closed or open fractures of the limbs treated in the "therapeutic village". Patients with or without X-ray cliche treated in the "therapeutic village" of ZE Kane; The nursing staff of the Adjap district medical centre (CMA).

VI.4. The film's characters

Our various stakeholders include two care staff from the "therapeutic village", patients and two sick callers.

VI .5. People interviewed outside the shoot

In the course of our research, we interviewed 35 people, including two village chiefs, 5 sick nurses, 6 elderly people and 25 patients, all of whom were willing to share their experiences of illness and care for patients with fractures, as well as their knowledge of traditional medicine.

VII . WRITING FILM PRODUCTION MATERIALS

This section includes the film's idea, synopsis, storyboard and sequences.

VII.1 Film idea

In everyday life, there are both happy and unhappy events, such as accidents that happen to individuals, causing physical trauma (fractures, sprains, dislocations, etc.) and leading people to seek treatment either in hospitals or, traditionally, from traditional healers in "therapeutic villages". Knowing that illness is a universal, each culture has developed its own explanations as to why we fall ill and, once we are ill, what we need to do to get better. Using our camera and an anthropological perspective on health, our work focuses on the link between the needs of the population and the health and care responses, and involves observing, analysing and understanding the rationale for directing patients to 'therapeutic villages' and how bone diseases are treated using endogenous therapeutic knowledge that is tending to disappear in our different communities.

VII.2 Synopsis

This is a presentation in words of a brief summary of the major part or point that will be shown in our film in relation to our research problem. An ethnographic film made by a visual anthropology student with the aim of observing, analysing and understanding fracture care practices and patients' impressions in a "therapeutic village". Filmed in Nko'olong in the Niete 2022 district. With the participation of ZE Kane Samuel, MONAYONG Martin, EYOMANE Christiane Desiree.

V II.3. The storyboard and film sequences

After composing the synopsis for the film, we drew up a storyboard, also known as a shooting guide. According to Warblefly (2020), the storyboard is an important element in the pre-production of a film, as it allows the storyline to be clearly explained. The aim of the story board is to classify the different sequences and the different shots that have been executed in each scene. We will also look at the different techniques used to develop the film, i.e. framing, camera movements, shooting angles, their timing, etc. (Cf. appendix). Based on the observations made in our area of exploration, we were able to reconstruct the care activities in the practice of bone disease care. The various care activities that make up the practice of bone disease care (bone fractures) include the following: Patient reception: the patient is admitted to the care unit, which is the "therapeutic village" in the form of a dormitory. If the patient has already had an X-ray, he or she is admitted to the treatment unit in the therapeutic village; if not, the patient is referred to a hospital for an X-ray. On his return, the traditherapeute analyses the X-ray images, consults the patient, locates the fracture and begins treatment. He begins by preparing the medicine, making the 'Akang'. Once these elements have been assembled, the actual treatment begins. Generally speaking, treatment takes place in the afternoon, with massage, scarification, application of the medicine, drying of the medicine, bandaging and local immobilisation, followed by rehabilitation and the armouring ritual. The table below will form our shooting guide. (see Appendix).

V   II. 4 The different sequences of the film

The film EKPWELE DOKITA BI-VE (The Bone Doctor's Incision) is a film based on our research theme: ZE Kane's therapeutic village: bone disease treatment practices in Niete. The film begins with a brief presentation of the "therapeutic village" using a tracking shot, followed by a presentation of the therapists ZE Kane and his son MONAYONG Martin. Medium shots are used. After this brief presentation, we show the process of making "ndoup" with the interaction of ethno-cinematographer and therapist and the preparation of the massage infusion. After preparing the medicine, the therapist devotes himself to making a tool for immobilising the fracture site, the 'akang'. A short transition shows the crossing of the bridge, as if to say that traditional medicine goes elsewhere to seek the best for its effectiveness.

This transition is followed by the restoration of patients and then the analysis of a patient's x-ray image by therapists. Here, traditional therapists discuss and analyse the patient's x-ray image. Once the image has been analysed, massage, scarification and the application of the drug 'ndoup' follow, while the therapist, patient and ethno-cineast interact.

Once the 'ndoup' has been applied, the traditional therapist immobilises the fracture site with a bandage and the 'Akang'. The film ends with the patient being re-educated, which immediately leads to a ritual of armouring, including the preparation of chicken and plantain, followed by a meal. The patient returns two weeks later to thank the therapist for his work.

V   II. 5 The film interview guide

We drew up a film interview guide that enabled us to interact with our informants. It was a set of questions drawn up after immersion that enabled me to gain a better understanding of the practice of caring for bone diseases.

This interview guide also shows the ethno-cineastes' involvement in the construction of the story they wish to tell (see appendix).

VII.6. Authorisations

We would like to remind you here that authorisations are papers or documents issued by an authority or senior official in the jurisdiction where we wish to carry out our research. This document covers the 'door' and protects the researcher in his field when he respects the stipulated steps of the research in whatever situation we find ourselves. Since our research is basic research, also known as academic research, an authorisation is first issued by our school (Attestation de Recherche); (see appendix) which proves that we are students and that we are fit to carry out research. In addition to this, we also have three (3) other forms of authorisation which will guide us in our work and we will tell you about the fagon from which we obtained the authorisations and signatures.

VII.7. Research authorisation.

This authorisation was intended for the highest authority in our study area, the sub-prefect of the Niete district. Before negotiating with our informants, we thought it would be a good idea to have a document from an authority in the area justifying us carrying out research in their area. We wrote a request to the sub-prefect with a copy of our national identity card, university fee receipts and our Research Certificate from the sociology/anthropology department. We then went to the relevant administration to hand in the documents on 17 November 2021. When we arrived, the first deputy looked us over and told us we had three days to collect the document. Three days later, the document had still not been delivered to be signed by the electricity company. After spending weeks, we had to wait until 10 December 2021, the date on which our document was issued, guaranteeing that we were fit to work on our research site (see appendix).

VII .8. Drawing up the shooting permit

As part of our work, we drew up a photography permit to submit to the Ocean departmental delegate for arts and culture. On November 2021 the departmental delegate issued us with the photographic licence (see Appendix).

VIII   9. Drawing up the authorisation to transfer rights

Before we could begin shooting and producing our film, we had to draw up an authorisation document for our actors, known as a "Contract for the transfer of rights". In French, it is known as the "Contrat de cession des droits". This document, although it covers the researcher, gives a limit to what we can and cannot do with the images and sound collected from our actors and informants (see appendix).

IX   II. SHOOTING EQUIPMENT

VIII.1 The Canon vixia HF R800 HD camcorder)

As part of our work, we used a Canon VIXIA HF R800 HD camcorder.

V   III.1.1. Advantages of the Canon Vixia HF R800 HD

With its powerful zoom, this tool lets you capture moments up close, far away and everywhere in between. Exciting features include Highlight Priority mode with backlight correction, which gives you the best possible shots, and enhanced slow-motion and fast-motion recording, which lets you experiment with new ways of shooting. The light weight of the CANON VIXIA HF R800 means you can keep it close at hand to shoot what you need to shoot when you need to shoot it. Removable SD memory cards provide a quick and convenient way to share footage.

V   III.1.2 Drawbacks of the Canon Vixia HF R800 HD

The device does not have an internal data storage capacity which makes the data collected from an SD card vulnerable to attack by viruses.

V   III.2 Drafting of tools for collecting data

In accordance with our research protocol, we used a number of tools to collect knowledge discourse. The filming guide for our interactions with the actors, the observation guide and the interview guide.

The interviews were conducted using a video camera for the filmed interviews and a mobile phone using the magnetophone application for the recordings, in the absence of a suitable dictaphone.

VIII.2.1. The interview guide

The interview guide is an important element in anthropological research; it seeks to show the unity of field research over and above the diversity of its tools. The interview guide orients the researcher, especially the apprentice anthropologist. In other words, direct or assisted administration to a population guarantees the researcher that only the people indicated are those who will respond to the survey. Unlike the distributed questionnaire which, apart from being easy to use and saving survey time, has flaws that are more or less the result of bias in rural Africa, the interview guide reassures the researcher that he is dealing with the target person.

This method enabled us to reassure the informants that we were complementary and easy to understand, so that they would not feel embarrassed if they had not answered correctly. The discussions focused on knowledge of the human body, disease, fractures, knowledge of pharmacopoeia and the reasons that determine the therapeutic choice of traditional medicine in the event of a bone fracture in a patient. We drew up five interview guides for our research. All these interviews took the form of semi-directive interviews.

VIII.2.2. Semi-structured interviews :

The individual interview is a research method that involves questioning a person orally. It is a face-to-face meeting with the informant. We therefore conducted semi-directive interviews with care staff from the therapeutic village, patients, elderly people and care staff from the Adjap CMA. The purpose of these interviews was to examine the perceptions, representations and interactions that take place in the therapeutic village, a space for socialisation.

VIII.2.3. The interview guide for patients

Our observations in the research field enabled us to draw up an interview guide for patients. This enabled us to understand the different reasons why patients come to therapeutic villages, their itineraries, their perceptions of traditional medicine and their interactions (see Appendix).

VIII. 2.4. Interview guide for therapists

This interview guide enabled us to understand bone disease care practices. It was administered to two health workers from the ZE Kane therapeutic village (see appendix).

III.2.5. Interview guide for public health staff

To contrast our data from the therapeutic village, we also questioned public health staff to understand the different reasons why certain patients may be brought to "therapeutic villages" (see Appendix).

VIII.2.6. The turning guide

It was a series of questions written up after immersion that helped me to better understand the practice of caring for bone diseases (see Appendix).

To contrast our data collected from our informants, we carried out direct observations and participant observations.

VIII.3 Direct observation :

It is a technique that involves systematic observation and recording of human behaviour or a phenomenon and aspects of the environments in which they occur in order to obtain specific information. This method enabled us to see first-hand how trauma patients are cared for - the preparation of medication, the manufacture of immobilisation tools, massage - in short, the entire process of caring for a patient suffering from bone disease.

VIII. 4. Life stories

Life stories have a strong capacity for intelligibility, as they help to bring out the meaning that individuals attribute to their actions, in particular by stimulating their reflective capacities. Through this research, we gathered personal experiences of a fracture situation: a 73-year-old patient who had already cared for her two children at ZE Kane's and who was the third patient in this family to suffer a fracture declared that "do we have anyone else?", the different therapeutic itineraries and experiences of the care practices of our informants. The effect of these life stories was to immerse us in the vision of our informants and to relive the situations that led them to the traditional treatment of fractures, and to the care practices in the therapeutic village of ZE Kane.

VIII.5. Participant observation :

Participatory observation is a term that refers to the fieldwork of the father of functionalist anthropology (Malinowski 1992). He conducted field research among the Melanesians for three and a half (03) years, which means that a researcher goes out into the field to immerse himself in reality, in order to get to know human beings, a knowledge that comes through communicating with them and sharing their existence in a lasting way. This immersion in the therapeutic village of ZE Kane gave us the opportunity to practise patient care activities, to participate in the treatment of patients by assisting therapists in their care practices and also by helping patients with their requests.

IX. ETHICAL INVOLVEMENT

It is about the impact and consequences that our research can have on an individual's right. As Lopez says in (2009:31)

"Ethics as a subset of normativity, to encompass rational discourses and practices whose aim is to systematise or formally reflect on the moral conduct or good behaviour of individuals".

The aim of this fundamental and academic research is to observe, understand and analyse care practices in the management of fractures in a "therapeutic village". This is a goal that social science researchers are striving to achieve in order to preserve local practices, cultures, knowledge and know-how, which are tending to disappear. Ethics in research is a set of rules designed to ensure that scientific activity is subject to respect for values deemed to be higher than the researcher's freedom.

As part of this project, we can anticipate certain sensitive issues that could affect our shoot by being objective about the different issues we want to tackle.

The aim was to seek out, detect and film what is not said in the practice of fracture care (gestures, positions, interactions, etc.) and to write about what is said, because there is a large body of literature on the practice of bone disease care.

We have tried to guarantee and preserve the interests of our informants by protecting the content of our project within the structures responsible for protecting audiovisual content. To avoid any form of misunderstanding, we have informed the administrative, security and traditional authorities in our research area. All other people likely to be involved in our film as a resource person through a correspondent, with the aim of raising their awareness and begging them to support us in the successful production of our film. As fundamental research in its own right, we looked for ways and means of involving our informants in the project of making our ethnographic film. This was achieved through mutual support between ethno-cineastes, traditional therapists and patients, and through the anonymity of our informants.

IX.1 Identification of risks

We will try to establish very good relations with our informants because by establishing good relations with the community, the community adopts you and this can contribute to your safety in the research field. We will obtain research authorisations from the school and then apply for authorisations from the administration in charge of arts and culture. These various authorisations will be submitted to the administrative, traditional and security authorities in our study area.

As far as our research is concerned, there are no particular problems associated with being a woman.

Similarly, for our travel security, we need to use travel agencies and avoid clandestine transport as much as possible. Given that the camera is our main tool in this search, we must do all we can to protect our equipment, i.e. be careful about where our luggage is deposited.

There is no particular risk to our health, but before we leave for our research field, we will be preparing a first-aid kit in case we feel unwell in the field.

X. PRODUCTION

This section looks at the various stages leading up to the production of our film.

X.1. Shooting time

Our film was shot over a period of three months at two locations: ZE KANE SAMUEL's "therapeutic village" and the Adjap district medical centre.

X.2.1 Problems and difficulties encountered

Our research was hampered by a number of difficulties:

From an administrative point of view, we did not receive the various authorisations we requested in time.

On a practical level, a lack of audio-visual equipment made our work difficult by prolonging our time in the field, and the fact that our study area was isolated in terms of communication and telecommunication also made our task difficult, as it was almost impossible to communicate with our supervisor while we were in the field.

Similarly, the reluctance of some of our informants, knowing that our theme dealt with issues of intimacy, therapeutic choice and health, made it difficult at first for them to allow us to move forward with our research. It took the intervention of the therapist and good immersion in the patients through my interest in them for them to agree to collaborate and take part in the study.

X.2.2 Interaction and empathy during filming

Many of the patients who arrive at the ZE KANE "therapeutic village" have been virtually abandoned by their families. Seeing men, women and children in suffering situations prompts us to take the necessary decisions to help these vulnerable people. As a result, throughout our time in the field, we established very good relations not only with the therapists, but also with all the patients in the "therapeutic village". As one of our informants put it

QMZ "And who looks after the upkeep of your sleeping area?"

RENP " Oh, we've had manna from heaven, we've had manna from heaven in the form of a young boy from this village who came for his studies, really, in the one and a half months I've been here, I'd never seen him before, but this young gareon has really brought clarity to the village, really, really it's been a great heart for him. A really big heart for us patients and for the tradi and his son. So it was this gareon who gave us a helping hand and we take our hats off to him and say a big thank you.

Our assistance consisted of tidying up around the compound, assisting the therapist in his care practices by starting to heat the pots each day before the massage, and carrying the feet of patients who didn't have sick shifts. We helped the patients by running errands, cleaning their belts and clothes, making water for washing and drinking, emptying the patients' pots and sometimes cooking for them. The evening of our departure was the day we felt all the suffering endured by patients suffering from bone diseases. After thanking them, we said a prayer, and it was at the end of our prayer that the suffering became apparent, as we cried for minutes thinking about the situation of these patients. A sign of a painful separation from my investigations.

XI. POST-PRODUCTION

Post-production is all the stages that precede production, i.e. the selection of rushes, the narrative framework and the organisation of the rushes in the software.

XI.1 Selection of rushes

The selection of rushes was based on the story of the "therapeutic village" that we wanted to tell.

In our various shots, we established daily shot-lists. These daily shot-lists enabled us to classify our hives by theme, which made it easier for us to tell the story.

XI.2 The narrative

The narrative framework is a way for the filmmaker to tell his or her film. From an anthropological and ethnographic perspective, the films resulting from this research are generally stories about reality, and as Mac Dougall (1978), quoted by Sardan, points out, '*you need a thread or a means of transport*'. Once we had come up with the idea for our film, we identified the different themes that we would develop in our work. Given that our subject deals with practices that obey a process, we wanted to tell the story of bone disease care practices in chronological order. Our film is built around three main parts: an introduction, a development and a conclusion. These different parts are separated from each other using transitional images from our filming area.

XI.3. Organisation of rushes in the software

Having established a narrative framework that would enable us to tell a story about bone disease care practices in ZE Kane's therapeutic village, we chose an editing software package (CyberLink PowerDirector) to build our story.

XII. THE THEORETICAL FRAMEWORK

In this part of my work, I will briefly describe the conceptual corpus (theories) in which this work is embedded and with which I will be "dialoguing" throughout my fieldwork. These concepts correspond point by point to a unit of understanding of individual orientation towards "therapeutic villages", namely: the concepts of : Representational dynamics, and the theory of observational cinema.

Our subject is part of a research approach in social and cultural anthropology, see the anthropology of health, whose perspective is the analysis and interpretation of the logics that direct patients towards endogenous know-how of traditional therapeutic care practices in the care of patients suffering from physical trauma, in particular (dislocation, rheumatism, bone fracture, sprain, dislocation, etc.).

The anthropology of health studies illness from the point of view of concepts and conception Fainzang (2000: 7) writes:

"In an attempt to define this new knowledge constituted by medical anthropology, we must first clear up a misunderstanding. This misunderstanding is that which consists in seeing this discipline as a branch of the medical sciences which would focus its attention on cultural conceptions of evil, with a view to helping health professionals in their task. Such a misunderstanding places medical anthropology on the fringes of what defines it as social and cultural anthropology, and prevents us from understanding how the approach to disease constitutes, for the anthropologist, an object of knowledge like any other.

The field of medical anthropology is generally understood to include research which focuses on representations of illness, the itineraries of patients, the role of therapists or therapeutic practices of all kinds (including healing rituals), in relation to the socio-cultural system in which they are embedded, health professionals and health care production companies. Research in medical anthropology has taken two main directions: functionalist and cognitive. In the functionalist direction, the main aim of this research has been to investigate the social function of representations of illness in the societies studied. The cognitive orientation focuses on the ways in which different cultures perceive and structure experience. It seeks to identify the categories forged by these cultures in order to understand the experience of illness. Our perspective is therefore to work in a traditional institution that offers therapeutic care to patients in a rural context, i.e. care practices for bone diseases (dislocation, bone fracture, sprain, dislocation, etc.).

In our context, a number of issues can be studied in the context of a 'therapeutic village', namely: the medical institution, the nursing staff, the relationship between the nurse and the patient, the drug, the patients' therapeutic itinerary, medical practices, the origin of medical knowledge, the disease, therapeutic effectiveness, beliefs and perceptions. In short, there are a number of themes that raise questions about the traditional medical institution that is the 'therapeutic village'. From a visual perspective, the theme that is most relevant to our topic here is the treatment of bone fractures.

XII.1 The theory of social representations

The dynamic concept of representation: The theory of "social" representations (TRS) was first developed by the psychologist Serge Moscovici in his 1961 study of psychoanalysis, for whom representation has both an individual and a social origin. Since then, it has been widely developed, first in Europe and then internationally. Moscovici (1961) follows in the footsteps of authors such as Freud, Piaget and Durkheim, from whom he drew inspiration in formalising the concept of social representation. Social representations (SR) are a set of opinions, information, values and beliefs about a particular object (the object of the representation). A "social representation is therefore always a representation of something (the object) and someone (the subject)". This object-group relationship is the principle around which the theory of social representations is organised.

Social representation' (SR) is a cross-disciplinary concept, situated at the interface of the psychological and the social, which makes its definition complex. For Moscovici, the founding father of social representation theory (SRT), it is: "a way of interpreting the world and thinking about our everyday reality, a form of social knowledge that people construct more or less consciously on the basis of what they are, what they have been and what they project, and which guides their behaviour. And correlatively (SR is) the mental activity deployed by individuals and groups to fix their positions in relation to situations, events, objects and communications that concern them" (Moscovici, 1984).

According to Jodelet (1997), representation: "is a form of knowledge that is socially elaborated and shared, has a practical purpose and contributes to the construction of a common reality for a social group. It is not a simple reflection of reality, but functions as a system for interpreting reality, organising the relationships between individuals and their environment and guiding their practices". Situated at the frontier between the psychological and the social, social representations enable individuals and groups to master their environment and act upon it.

Jean-Claude Abric (1997) defines "social representation" as "a functional vision of the world, which enables the individual or group to give meaning to their behaviour, and to understand reality, through their own system of reference, and thus to adapt to it and define their place within it". For Roussiau and Bonardi (2001): "A social representation is an organisation of socially constructed opinions, relative to a given object, resulting from social communications, making it possible to master the environment and to appropriate it on the basis of symbolic elements specific to the group or groups to which one belongs".

A social representation is therefore an "object" shared between a "me" (the ego) and "the others" (the alter). It is a universe of opinions shared by a group and developed through communication. It reflects the individual experiences and social practices of individuals. Representation enables us to understand and act on the world.

It is a concept that enables us to grasp the social realities of individuals, which in turn enables us to solve certain social problems and construct psychological representations. Social representation is a concept that came into its own in French universities, particularly at the Ecole des Hautes Etudes in Paris and the psychology department in Marseille. Firstly, under the leadership of Serge Moscovici (1961), who was the first to take up the idea already formulated by E. Durkheim when he introduced the term 'collective representation' in his work on 'suicide', and popularised it by giving it a social dimension. In fact, when he wanted to find out what the French public thought about psychoanalysis, he showed, or rather he discovered, that not everyone knew about it. Some people (students, teachers, professionals), because of their proximity to psychoanalysis, were able to talk about it at length, while others (workers) had no knowledge of it and could not give it a dimension that would enable them to understand it in an exhaustive or even approximate way. Domo Joseph, analysing the relations of the representational dynamics between the Chad/Cameroon riparian populations, writes:

"People living along the river, and even those living inland, can discern the nature of relations between Cameroon and Chad from an individual perspective. The closer one is to the sphere, where contacts are frequent, the more likely one is to perceive the issues from a much more global angle. On the other hand, remoteness is a reducing factor, except for those who, professionally or for any other reason, are likely to have a better grasp of the socio-economic reality in force".

Moscovici has opened a door that is not about to close again. Since then, it has been a real stimulus for research, especially in social psychology. Studies have been undertaken in order to arrive at the conceptualisation of one or more tools capable of providing proof of the facts. This is what Claude Flament cited by Domo Joseph, It was Claude Flament, quoted by Domo Joseph, who in 1973 operationalised the instrument of a technique to try to resolve this area of uncertainty which led some to say that the social sciences are soft sciences as opposed to hard sciences, i.e. all those which base their existence on figures, This is how he developed the analysis of similarity, which makes it possible to visualise the relationships that exist between two elements, but above all to read through a graffiti the maximum tree of correspondences between the different constituent elements, for example, in our context, to evaluate the supply of biomedical care in relation to the supply of traditional practices, phytotherapists, in short, traditional medicine.

J.C Abric in turn introduced another notion, that of the central core. All social representations are built around a central element, the core, which gives weight and meaning to the whole representation. It resists change, and it is because of this characteristic that the representation remains what it is, i.e. stable, not subject to the upheavals that can occur at any time. The representation therefore resists and retains its meaning as long as the structure of this core is not shaken: it is therefore the peripheral elements that move and change. When we speak of the transformation of a representation, we mean the destruction of its entire internal structure, and to achieve this, it takes the emergence of very special situations of great scope to bring about such a transformation, such an upheaval.

People from the 1 arrondissement of Niete and elsewhere come to ZE KANE Samuel's "therapeutic village" because they find solutions to their problems of bone disease, particularly bone fractures. They have therefore built an idea around the "central core", which is the practice of treating bone diseases in this therapeutic village.

XII.2 The theory of observational cinema

The theory of observational cinema is the characteristic approach of anthropological films today. In fact, the concern in observational cinema is to find the truth. Here, it's a question of provoking the real from the hidden by building trust with your research (immersion). Similarly, the ethno-filmmaker must respect certain principles:

Open your mouth to sensitive issues by creating themes beforehand (interview guide, filming guide, etc.)

Make the audiovisual tool (Camera) appear consciously by letting the interviewer see what he wants to show or is used to doing without adding any role whatsoever,

Based on long shots

Other approaches need to be taken into account, such as the theory of the informant's voice-over taken during an interview, the talking silent image, confining the film to the audience or allowing the informants to converse (subtitling).

Linked to our scientific undertaking, this conceptual and theorical framework remains very important in analysing and understanding the practices and orientations or individual therapeutic choices made by individuals in their different environments. This is why the whole of this theorical and conceptual framework enabled us to make analytical choices based on the data collected from our informants.

XIII. Work plan

Our work is structured and segmented into four main chapters: chapter one presents the study area, chapter two presents the therapeutic village and its characteristics. Chapter three describes the practice of treating bone diseases and the fourth chapter analyses the representations and perceptions of traditional medicine and the interactions of the therapeutic village.

CHAPTER I

PRESENTATION OF THE STUDY AREA
INTRODUCTION

The Arrondissement de la Commune de Niete is an agro-industrial zone located in the south of Cameroon near the Atlantic coast in the Ocean Department. The anthropological approach to research requires the researcher to master his or her working space. In the context of our study of ZE KANE Samuel's 'therapeutic village': practices in the care of o. gonorrhea diseases, it is important to present our findings. For this, it is important to briefly present our study area in order to know and situate our work in time and space. We therefore thought it would be useful to highlight the essential aspects of our study area, which is the district of Niete. This chapter will enable us to give an organisational overview of our environment, then present the geographical location and finally the assets and potential of this area.

1. The organisation

In addition to the Hevecam plantation, the Commune d'Arrondissement of Niete includes the following villages: Adjap, Afan oveng, Akom I, Bidou III, Bifa, Ngog, Nko'olong, Nkolmbonda and Zingui. The Niete district has a chiefdom of 2^e degree and 836 Bulu groups. Following the four cardinal points, the communes bordering the Niete arrondissement include: to the north, the commune of Lokoundje, to the north-east the commune of Lokoundje, to the north-west the commune of Lokoundje, to the south the commune of Campo, to the south-east the commune of Campo, to the south-west the commune of Kribi 1er , to the east the commune of Akom II, and to the west the commune of Lokoundje.

Our research will focus specifically on the village of Nko'olong, where ZE KANE Samuel, a traditional practitioner, treats bone fractures.

1.1. Geographical location of the study area

The commune of Niete was created by decree N° 95/082 of 24 April 1995 creating the rural commune of Niete. The commune of Niete has a population of 40,894 spread over 28 villages covering an area of 2,117 km2. It is located in the South region, in the Ocean department, on the border with the North.

The first village at the western entrance to the Commune (Nkolmbonda) is about twenty kilometres from the town of Kribi. The Commune lies between the UTM coordinates 292000N - 632000E and 324000N - 636000E.

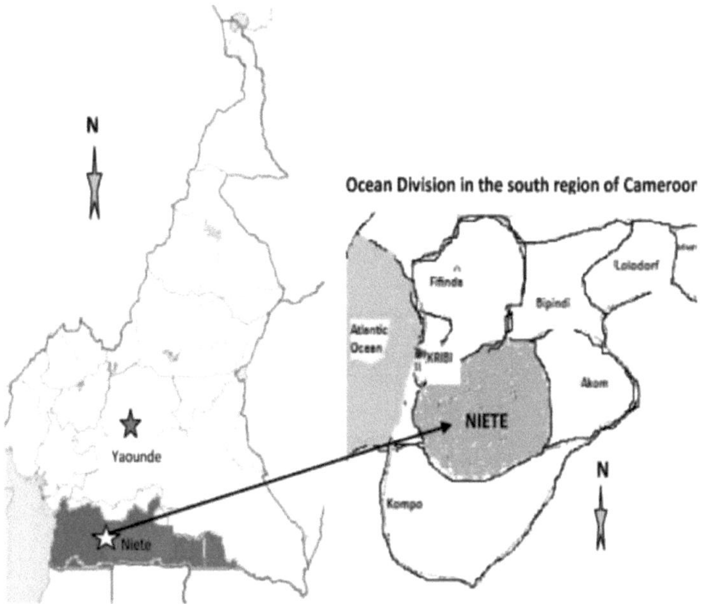

Map 1: Location of the district of Niete
Source: CVUC

1.2. The biophysical environment

The biophysical environment of the district of Niete is made up of the following geographical elements: climate, soil, relief and hydrography.

1.3. The climate

The prevailing climate in the district of Niete is equatorial Guinean, with four seasons: A long dry season starting from November to mid-March; a short rainy season starting from mid-March to mid-June; a short dry season starting from mid-June to mid-August and finally a long rainy season starting from mid-September to November. The average temperature over the course of a year is 25°C, humidity is 75% per year and rainfall varies between 1800 and 2000 mm per year.

1.4. Soils

The Commune d'arrondissement of Niete has two main types of soil: ferralitic soils and hydro-morphic soils. The more common ferralitic soils, used for agriculture, are relatively poor, requiring amendments for intensive farming or prolonged fallow periods to allow the soil to recover.

The hydro-morphic soils, which are less widespread, are used for off-season crops along wetlands and riverbanks.

1.5. The relief

The relief throughout the Niete commune is relatively flat within the hevevcam plantation, forming a plateau at altitudes of between 20 and 200 metres. The relief of the rural area is uneven, with elevations of up to 300 metres along the rivers.

1.6. HYDROGRAPHY

The district of Niete is located in the Atlantic Basin, and is crossed by the Kienke and Lobe rivers, as well as a number of other watercourses, most notably the Tyangue and Niete. The Niete runs alongside the Hevecam plantation, through the urban centres of village 2 (V2) and village 7 (V7), before emptying into the Lobe at village 15 (V15). The Kienke flows northwards through the villages of Adjap, Akom I, Nko'olong and Nkolmbonda, forming a natural boundary with the Commune of Lokoundje.

1.7. Flora and fauna

The vegetation of the commune of Niete is that of the dense equatorial forest, hydrophilic and evergreen. However, secondary and primary forests can be found as one moves away from the settlements and towards the interior of the forest. It is in these different forests of the district that traditherapeutes penetrate to find the essential elements that make up the remedy needed to treat their patients. The main forest species in the district are presented in a table in the appendix.

The municipality also boasts a wide variety of fauna, some of which are listed in a table in the appendix.

1.8. The human environment

Written and individual sources have enabled us to describe the human environment, populations, relations between ethnic groups, religions, economic activities and health structures.

1.9. Historical landmarks

The commune of Niete was created by decree No. 95/082 of 24 April 1995 creating the rural commune of Niete. In order to bring the administrators closer to the people of Hevecam, the government found it imperative to create the District of Niete by decree N°92/187 of 1er September 1992. By decree N°2010/198 of 16 June 2010, the District of Niete became the Arrondissement of Niete, with Adjap as its administrative centre. The administrative unit of Niete has now been relocated to Adjap. The district has now had its third sub-prefect and its second mayor since the administrative unit was created.

1.10.   The population

The Commune d'Arrondissement of Niete has around 40894 inhabitants spread across 28 villages. According to the Niete communal development plan (PCDN), the communal population is made up of 19137 men, 11154 women, 5655 young people aged 05-16 and 4948 young people under 5. The population of the Hevecam plantation zone is estimated at 25,437, or 62.20% of the total population. Of this total population, there are around 3,400 Baguyeli. The Baguyeli represent only 1.85% of the total population of the Commune.

1.11.   The local Bulu and Baguyeli populations

The Bulu are a Bantu-speaking people living in southern Cameroon and forming part of the "Sanaga-Ntem complex", a larger ethnic group that also includes the Beti and Fang - referred to as "Pahouins" by most French writers since the beginning of the century.

The district of Niete comprises ten Bulu villages adjacent to the HEVECAM plantation, known as the "groupement Bulu Sud". These villages form ten "traditional chiefdoms" (known as 3eme degree chiefdoms), each corresponding to a village. Heading east-west, we find the Bulu chiefdoms of Nkolmbonda, Bidou III, Nko'olong, Nlozok, Andjek, Angalle, Akom I, Adjap, Zingui and Bifa. There are four main Bulu tribes in the present-day district: the Yemeyema (now in Bidou III, Nko'olong and Akom I), the Yessok (in Adjap), the Yemon (in Zingui and Bifa), and the Essakotan (in Nkolmbonda, Andjek and Angalle). These different communities are supervised by a group chieftaincy of the Southern Bulu (known as the 2[eme] degree chieftaincy) located at Zingui.

The arrival of the Bulu in Cameroon is relatively recent and has given rise to various hypotheses (see Alexandre, 1958; Laburthe-Tolra, 1981; Vansina, 1990). They are thought to have come from Upper Egypt and to be related to the Zande of Upper Ubangi. From the 18th century onwards, they left the savannah, probably under pressure from the Peul, and crossed the Sanaga river. They then moved steadily south-westwards through the forest. Their adaptation to this new environment was a crucial element in their changing culture; their progress was never a rapid march but rather a slow swarming of villages. The constant direction of their migration has been explained by religious motives (the sunset is in fact the land of their ancestors that they wished to return to) or economic motives (the commercial centres on the coast).

Migration came to an end at the end of the 19th century, halted by the colonial administration. The Bulu were quickly Christianised and educated, with the result that a large proportion of Cameroon's first elites (working in the colonial administration in particular) were Bulu, such as the current president Paul Biya or, at the other extreme if you like, the writer Mongo Beti. Yet many rural Bulu continue to pursue a traditional way of life based on agricultural use of the forest and forest products. The forest appears to be a domain that human beings use to satisfy their needs, gradually and sparingly. The Bulu practise itinerant agriculture over open fields (cassava, bananas, yams, oil palm, groundnuts). The chiefdoms of Andjek and Angalle are grouped together under the name Afan-Oveng.

Each family produces what it needs by growing its own crops. A typical family field covers an area of 0.3 to 1.5 hectares and is farmed for around 2 consecutive years, while fallow land lasts from 3 to 10 years, but sometimes much longer. Hunting, fishing and gathering still provide a central part of the diet.

Cash crops (cocoa, coffee, hevea latex, palm oil) are currently a major source of income. The human habitat consists of a family's huts, courtyard, domestic animals and fruit trees. The house is occupied by a man and his wife (or wives), their children, and the wives of sons and grandsons. A series of houses makes up a hamlet, and a series of hamlets makes up a village.

Photo 2: Houses built

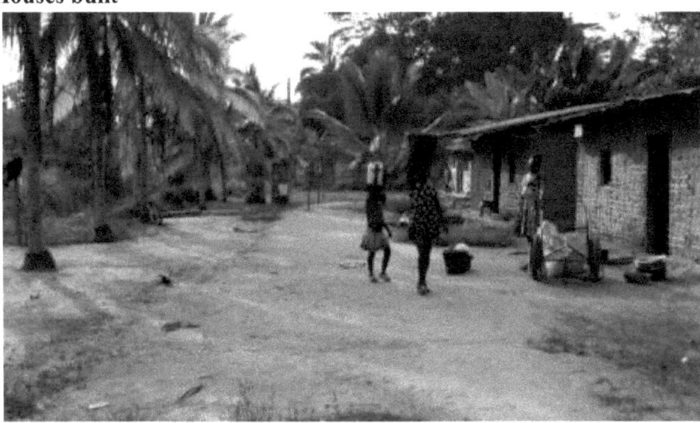

Source : *image du terrain photo Meric Zongo le 11 Decembre 2021 Nko 'oOng " village therapeutique*

The Arrondissement of Niete also includes four Baguyeli "Pygmy" communities, again following a north-south axis: Ngola, in (Nko'olong) Nkol- Ekoug, (located in Adjap), Bomlafenda, and Nyamabande. (Located in Nkolmbonda). The Baguyeli, also known as Bakola, are estimated to number around 3,400 people. They are located in the Ocean Department and in the north-west of Equatorial Guinea. The Baguyeli are thought to have originated in the Congo Basin, migrating to this region around the middle of the 19th century (Alexandre & Njomkap, 1998). The Baguyeli, like all hunter-gatherer peoples, are traditionally characterised by their lack of spatial anchorage and their remarkable mastery of space (Biesbrouck, 1999). Almost absolute dependence on the forest is the best-known reason for the semi-nomadism of the 'Pygmy' peoples, but mobility can also be explained, depending on the case, by the death of a relative, demographic pressure in a camp, competition for access to women, or the avoidance of internal and external conflicts.

Baguyeli communities (or bands) are structured around camps, which constitute the basic socio-economic environment. This is the place from which production/consumption activities are organised, based on hunting and gathering, but also, increasingly, on agriculture (including cash crops such as cocoa). A few huts (sometimes around ten), inhabited by a population that can vary from 15 to 70 people, generally relatives and allies from different exogamous clans, make up the community, which operates on a remarkably egalitarian basis.

1.12.   The cohabitation of the Bulu and Baguyeli peoples

The relationship between the Baguyeli and the Bulu (or, more generally, between the various Pygmy groups and the Bantu) developed from the moment they met through a series of exchanges of products and services: food crops, salt, iron tools and pottery on the part of the Bantu; hunting products, honey and medicines on the part of the Pygmy. These exchanges were reinforced by the attachment of Pygmy groups to Bantu clans as part of a symbolic kinship. Before colonisation, therefore, Bantu-Pygmy relations were based on reciprocity, but colonial demand for specific forest products (ivory, rubber, etc.), traditionally little valued by the Pygmy populations, meant that the Pygmy peoples had to make do with each other. - But the colonial demand for specific forest products (ivory, rubber, etc., traditionally little valued by the local populations), the obligation to pay taxes and the need for space for the new cocoa cultivation favoured the creation of a balance of power in favour of the Bantu: the Bantu-"Pygmy" relationship was then transformed into a relationship of sovereignty, and the latter still find themselves politically very marginalised.

The positions of 'chiefs' among the Bulu and Baguyeli were created from scratch by the colonial administration, which sought to use them as intermediaries and community leaders. It was also in this context that the forced sedentarisation of the Bantu and Pygmy peoples along the roads took place, as part of colonial and post-colonial policies aimed at improving control over the subjugated populations: the so-called traditional chiefdoms were thus created. In the Arrondissement of Niete, the Bulu and Baguyelis populations are unanimous.

1.13.   Religions

There are four main religions in the district of Niete. Christians, Muslims, Buddhists/Hindus and Animists. Among the Christians, there are three main denominations. The traditional churches, the Jehovah's Witnesses and the so-called revivalist churches:

As for Christian denominations, there are six main Protestant churches, including the Eglise Presbyterienne Camerounaise (EPC), the Eglise Presbyterienne Camerounaise Orthodoxe (EPCO), the Eglise Evangelique du Cameroun (EEC), the Eglise Jean Baptiste du Cameroun (EJBC), the Eglise Adventiste du Cameroun (EAC) and the Congregation Baptiste du

Cameroun (CBC), which is currently being established.

These are found in almost every village in the Commune, and their followers include the majority of the Commune's indigenous Bulu population. The EPC alone accounts for almost 60% of Protestant believers among the Bulu of Niete, followed by the EPCO (30%). The other four represent around 10%, and there is also a high proportion of Protestants on the plantation. 30% of HEVECAM's workers claim to belong to one of these denominations. Protestants therefore represent around 40% of the population of the Niete commune.

The Roman Catholic Church The Roman Catholic Church draws around 15% of its followers from the indigenous population of Niete. It also has a good proportion of the HEVECAM workers' community, also around 15%. The 15% of the commune's communities are therefore Catholic.

Jehovah's Witnesses: Jehovah's Witnesses (JWs) have their main followers (95%) in the HEVECAM workers' community. 5% of the indigenous population also identify with this religious denomination. We can therefore estimate a figure of 5% Jehovah's Witnesses in Niete.

The revivalist churches HEVECAM has two branches of revivalist churches:

The Pentecostal Church (EP) and the Apostolic Church (EA). They are mainly based in the HEVACAM plantation area, where they draw the majority of their followers from among the concession workers. Around 65% of HEVECAM's workers are in the Revivalist churches. There are so many variants of these denominations that they cannot all be mentioned: three in particular stand out: The English-speaking Pentecostal Church; the French-speaking Pentecostal Church; the Apostolic Church and the MARANATHA Pentecostal Church (EPM). 30% of the population of the commune of Niete belong to the Revivalist churches.

Muslims: The majority of Muslims are from North Cameroon and belong to the BAMOUN ethnic group. There are around 4% of Muslims in Hevecam, where they practise their faith at the mosque in village 07 of Hevecam (V7).

Animists Animism is found only among all the Pygmy communities (BAGUYELI) and a good number of "KIRDI" nationals from the far north, most of whom are employed as labourers by HEVECAM. This means that around 5% of HEVECAM's nationals are animists.

Buddhists/Hindus: Most of the Asian nationals who own HEVECAM-GMG are Buddhists. Buddhism is the religion of excellence in their country of origin, and they have no official representation or place of worship for their beliefs. The rites and celebrations of their beliefs are carried out solely at home. 1% of Niete's nationals are Buddhists.

1.14. The culture

Throughout the commune, there is virtually no place for cultural expression. There are only a few facilities belonging to the cultural associations of people from other parts of the country, such as the cultural hut for people from Bandjoun and the palaver hut for people from the South-West, both of which are located in village 7 (V7) of the plantation. In the rest of the commune, there has been a loss of cultural values due to the lack of cultural infrastructure, the absence of inter-generational dialogue, which has contributed to the disappearance of a good number of practices and dances (Mbaya, Tourne, etc.); the irregularity of cultural events, which have been replaced by extroversion and the depravation of local culture, crime, and a lack of tourist appeal to capitalise on the commune's cultural heritage. However, there are plans to implement cultural activities (1 fair a year), but these have not yet found a way to get off the ground, such as the construction of a cultural centre in Baguyelis, support for the dissemination of cultural heritage and the local know-how of the commune's communities.

1.15. Economic activities

The main economic activity is agriculture. Hevea cultivation is widespread in the commune, and is supplemented by other activities such as livestock rearing, small-scale trade, handicrafts and hunting. In general, subsistence farming is practised in the rural area by village populations.

Agriculture: this is practised by men, women and young people. The men grow hevea, oil palm, cocoa and plantain. Women grow food crops such as maize, cassava and yams. Baguyelis grow subsistence crops around their camps.

Breeding: on the hevecam plantations, employees breed pigs in pens. The villagers in the rural area and the Baguyelis practise traditional livestock farming.

Forestry: there has been an increase in the unregulated sawing of forest species, the search for firewood and the use of these forest resources for food and medical purposes.

Hunting: big game hunting takes place in and around Campo Ma'an and traditional hunting in the rural area.

Commerce: shops, drinking establishments, small subsistence businesses and the sale of non-timber forest products are the main commercial activities in the commune. At the end of each month, a regular market is held at Nlongo in the Hevecam plantation, where people from the rural area and the plantation buy supplies.

Handicrafts: the people of the Niete district commune thrive on basketry and the manufacture of fishing nets.

Banking services: the commune's financial flow is driven by microfinance institutions such as express unions, MC2, the post office, tontines and profit-making meetings.

Transport: transport is provided by motorbike taxis and clandos. Access to some localities is difficult due to a lack of suitable roads, which increases the number of accidents involving two-wheeled vehicles.

1.16. Healthcare facilities

Health concerns are dealt with by various state, religious and traditional health structures. The district chief town has an unequipped district medical centre (CMA), and a shortage of medical staff covers the entire rural area and part of the Akom II commune, with three health centres (Akok, Akom I and Zingui). The plantation area has a hospital and a church health centre. The reference hospital for the Adjap CMA is the Kribi district hospital. Access to quality health care is difficult due to poor infrastructure, a lack of pharmaceutical products, insufficient and specialised health care staff, poverty and the loss of human life, all of which lead to recourse to traditional pharmacopeia (therapeutic villages) and street medicines in many cases.

CONCLUSION

To sum up, this chapter is about presenting our zone.

of study by situating it on the national map of Cameroon. The Niete Arrondissement is a cosmopolitan commune with a wide range of assets and potential, whose curiosity is of interest to many researchers in various fields. Illness being a universal fact, we are therefore called upon to observe practices in a traditional health structure that offers care to patients suffering from bone diseases when cases of bone fractures occur. And the "therapeutic village" of ZE KANE, as the only specialised traditional health structure offering care to patients suffering from fractures in the Niete district, is a case to be observed from an anthropological angle. This presentation of our study area allows us to circumscribe our study in space and time to allow us to better deploy ourselves.

CHAPTER II

ZE KANE'S THERAPEUTIC VILLAGE

INTRODUCTION

The WHO defines traditional medicine as comprising various health practices, approaches, knowledge and beliefs incorporating plant-, animal- and/or mineral-based medicines, spiritual treatments, manual techniques and exercises, applied alone or in combination to maintain well-being, treat, diagnose or prevent disease. Traditional medicine has an important place alongside modern medicine in the treatment of bone diseases in Cameroon. It is closely linked to the socio-cultural world and is deeply rooted in the customs of Cameroonian society. The medical aspects of traditional medicine are broadly similar to those of modern medicine. It makes diagnoses, provides care and treatment and gives advice. In view of the many complications that result, it is important for us to look at the work carried out by ZE Kane and his son MONAYONG Martin, to see how bone diseases are treated. Although the WHO has been implementing a strategy since 2002 to integrate traditional medicine into national healthcare systems, this practice is still illegal and poorly understood in our country. Similarly, the texts relating to research on individuals have not been promulgated, which makes research on individuals difficult. ZE KANE Samuel's "therapeutic village", a specialist bone repair unit, treats several types of fracture or bone disease. This chapter presents this traditional health unit and how it works.

II. Presentation and location of the ZE KANE therapeutic village

The ZE KANE traditional healthcare unit (therapeutic village) is a traditional healthcare unit specialising in the repair of trauma (bone diseases: dislocation, sprain, dislocation fracture, etc.). The facility is located in Nko'olong. It's a village in the Niete Arrondissement in the Ocean Department, South Cameroon Region. Leaving Kribi, you take the road to Akom II. The village of Nko'olong is located 19 km from the town of Kribi on the road before the Hevecam SA junction. The building was constructed some thirty years ago and has a capacity of eight to ten patients. The building is made of rammed earth and is subdivided into two compartments, one of which is a dormitory or space reserved for patients, while the other serves as a kitchen for patients' meals. Inside the building, the dormitory beds are arranged in two rows, each with four beds per row. The beds are less than one metre apart. On arrival, patients choose the bed on which they will spend the rest of their stay. Patients do not have enough space and tables for their belongings. These belongings are usually also placed on the patients' beds. The kitchen area has cooking utensils and food supplies for patients. The tradi-therapist has provided his patients with everything they need, such as basins and buckets for storing water. Outside the building, a large courtyard separates the therapist's living room from the patient reception area. This courtyard is planted with coconut trees, which patients can pick as they please, as our informant put it: *"It's not good for your stranger to go and ask for what you've got"*.

Photo 3: *ZE Kane therapeutic village*

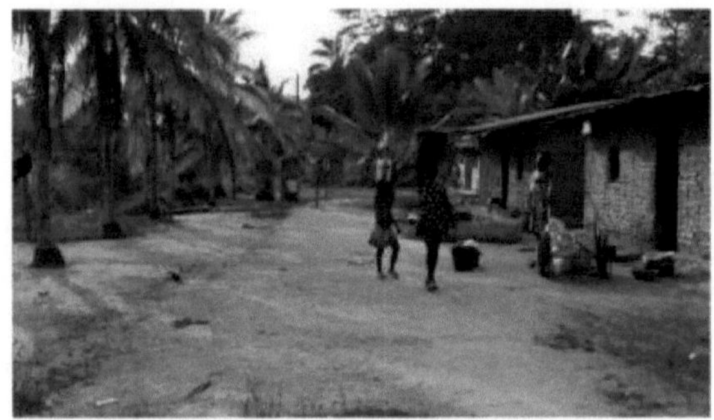

Source : *photo Meric Zongo le 11 Decembre 2021 Nko'olong " village therapeutique.*
At the back of the building is a cocoa plantation with other fruit trees such as avocado and mango, as well as a toilet block inside the cocoa plantation.

Map 2: Location of the therapeutic village in the Niete district

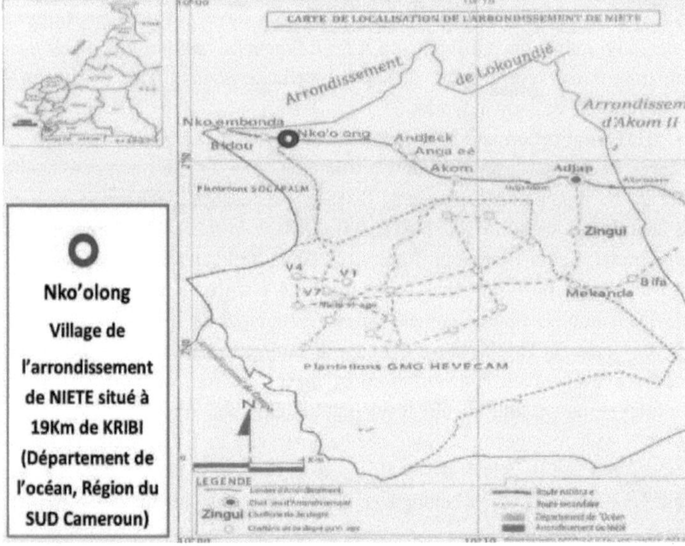

Source: CVUC

II.1 The structure of the therapeutic village

The building was constructed some thirty years ago. It's a mud building divided into two compartments, one of which is a dormitory or space reserved for patients, while the other serves as a kitchen for patients' meals.

1.1.1. . The interior

Inside the building, the dormitory area is divided into two rows of beds, with four beds in each row. The beds are less than one metre apart. On arrival, patients choose the bed on which they will spend the rest of their stay. Patients do not have enough tables for their belongings. These belongings are generally also placed on the patients' beds.

The kitchen area has cooking utensils and food storage for patients. The therapist provides his patients with everything they need, such as bowls and buckets for storing water, and pots and plates for eating.

П.1.2. The exterior

The outside of the structure in front is a large courtyard which separates the therapist's living room and the structure which receives patients. This courtyard is planted with coconut trees, which patients can pick as they please, because, as our informant says, "it's *not good for your stranger to go and ask for what you have"*.

Behind the structure is a cocoa grove with other fruit trees such as avocado and plum, and a toilet block inside the cocoa grove.

11.2. Welcoming patients

The ZE KANE bone disease treatment unit or "therapeutic village" receives two types of patient, whose itinerary varies depending on the disease and the treatment provided. In fact, there are two types of patient: documented patients and undocumented patients.

11.2.1. The reception area

The patient who has arrived introduces himself or herself or the members accompanying him or her. If the patient has certain documents to present, such as a medical document or a prescription, he or she presents them to the therapist, who asks questions about the period of the trauma.

11.3. Types of bone disease

The traditional trauma unit at ZE Kane specialises in the treatment of diseases affecting the bone. Whatever the type and structure of the trauma, patients can be treated using the therapeutic properties of the medicinal plants used in the ZE Kane therapeutic village. The patients who arrive are victims of fractures, sprains, dislocations and dislocations. In short, they are patients whose bodies have suffered a shock or trauma that requires therapeutic intervention. In ZE Kane's "therapeutic village", traumatic fractures are the most common lesions, firstly because of the acute and noisy nature of the trauma, which leads patients to consult a traditional therapist most often immediately after the trauma. Traumatic lesions can therefore have a favourable spontaneous evolution, leading patients to believe, rightly or wrongly, in the therapist's effectiveness. These lesions are highly varied, particularly in cases where the diagnosis is obvious or the patient presented with X-ray images, such as articular fractures, extra-articular fractures, dislocations and sprains. As a result, therapists can see all types of musculoskeletal conditions, from the simplest to the most serious. Traumatic lesions were mainly in the limbs, with a higher percentage in the lower limbs. In the course of our study, we found that injuries to the lower limbs mainly involved the leg and tibia, as a result of accidental falls and carelessness on the public highway, which accounted for a large proportion of patients who consulted GPs. As regards laterality, the right side was the most affected, which corresponds to the general population, the majority of whom are right-handed in our country. The table below summarises the 23 cases of trauma and the lesion sites of the patients who received treatment at the ZE Kane therapeutic village during the period covered by our study.

1.1.1. . Dislocation

Dislocation: Loss of contact between joint surfaces. Dislocation, commonly known as dislocation, is the complete dislocation of a joint. This trauma is characterised by a loss of contact between the two surfaces: the bones that form the joint are completely separated. When the loss of contact is partial, we speak of subluxation.

Dislocation can be accompanied by trauma to the ligaments or cartilage of the joint, leading to instability or arthrosis. In general, dislocations occur in several places: the shoulder, knee, elbow, hand, hips and finger joints. They are caused by traumatic shock: often during combat or gymnastic sports activities, accidental falls and repeated instability or subluxation in the same person. The characteristic determination can be summed up as follows: a sharp pain in the joint, a snapping sensation at the moment of trauma, an inability to use the joint. The shock then causes the patient to become sensitive to touch, and the joint is deformed, twisted or displaced, with a discolouration or sometimes a loss of sensation in the patient. During our research, three patients suffered ligament dislocations. One in the right knee, one in the left ankle and one in the left thumb.

1.1.2. . Sprain

Ligament distension or tearing, absence of bone displacement. Generally speaking, it is a painful lesion caused by ligament elongation or tearing. According to the Larousse French dictionary, it refers to a traumatic injury to a joint resulting from its sudden distortion, with stretching (mild sprain) or rupture (severe sprain) of the ligaments. According to the medical dictionary, it is a traumatic joint lesion caused by the sudden distortion of a joint (without any lasting displacement of the joint surfaces), accompanied by elongation or tearing of the ligaments. For us, a sprain occurs when the ligaments that attach one bone to another can be torn at the joints. We recorded one case during our time in the field. The patient in question was EVE'E JEAN YVES.

1.1.3. . Sprain

According to the medical dictionary, it is a violent and accidental distension of the ligaments (a ligament is a kind of cable that joins two pieces of bone forming a joint, and thus helps to stabilise it) of a joint.

1.1.4. . Fractures

A fracture or fracture fracture can be seen as a break in the bone or hard cartilage, most often as a result of direct or indirect trauma (impact, fall, torsion). Classified as a trauma of accidental origin, the WHO defines it as a complication of osteoporotic disease which may be simple (closed) when the bone is not exteriorised by the trauma or exposed (open) when the injury has torn away the tissue covering the bone or when one of the fragments of the broken bone pierces the skin, which varies according to the impact and the individual following a trauma or, more rarely, following a pathology where it may crack or break into several segments. According to the Micro Robert cited by TCHOUMI (2021), a fracture is a break in a bone or in the earth's crust. Bone fractures include several etiological signs that can be grouped into two types:

Traumatic fractures: these are the most common fractures caused by everyday activities.

Pathological fractures: these are fractures that occur when the bone is weakened (osteoporosis, osteolytic fractures).

In both cases, they have very different characteristics and evolve in very different ways, depending on their location and situation in the bone itself. Depending on the mechanism by which they occur, fractures may be the result of direct trauma: caused by falls, shocks, impacts of aggression, or indirect trauma, which is caused either by torsion or compression... And can have other lesions above or below (sprain). Fatigue fractures very often occur following repeated stresses on the bones. They are common in metastases and are most often seen in major sportsmen and women. However, they can only be confirmed by a bone scan.

11.4. Fracture mechanisms

During the course of this study, we noted that there are two mechanisms of traumatic fractures:

Direct mechanism: this occurs when the bone is broken on impact. The trauma first affects the peripheral soft tissues (in particular the skin covering), which can be severely damaged (especially in the case of crushing).

Indirect mechanism: the bone gives way at a distance from the point of application of the trauma, which causes compression, flexion or torsion of the bone, depending on the case (e.g. elbow fracture following a fall onto the wrist; leg fracture, with the foot locked to the ground and the lower limb twisted on its axis). In these conditions, soft tissue damage is less severe. In general, a fracture is defined by its site, the fracture lines, the number of fragments and their displacement. The site of the fracture: First of all, its identity, for example (fracture of the clavicle, fracture of the femur, fracture of the peroneum and, more precisely, its location in the bone: diaphyseal fracture (for example in the middle or lower third), metaphyseal or epiphyseal fracture and, in this case, the fracture may be articular or extra-articular, apophyseal fracture.

The fracture line: It is rarely incomplete, affecting only one cortical bone (e.g. green wood fracture in children: one cortical bone is broken, the other is simply inflected). It is most often complete, involving both cortices and separating the fragments. Simple fracture: bi-fragmentary fracture, the line is single and separates the two fragments, one proximal, the other distal. It may be oblique or spiral: the contact surface between the two separated fragments is larger, but they slide more easily over each other (unstable fracture).

The complex multi-fragmentary fracture: This is defined by several fracture features such as the tri-fragmentary fracture (example: tibial fracture with a 3rd small "butterfly wing" fragment) observed in one of our informants through his cliche. Similarly, a double-stage fracture: the two upper and lower fractures isolate an intermediate fragment, which often has inadequate blood supply. Multi-fragmentary fractures involve 4 or 5 fragments or more (comminuted fracture). The fragments are very numerous and small, and surgical reconstruction of the bone jigsaw is impossible.

Displacement of fragments: Fractures without displacement are rare

Displacement of diaphyseal fractures: angulation in the frontal plane (valgus, varus) or sagittal plane (recurvatum, flexum). Translation in the frontal plane (medial, lateral) or sagittal plane (anterior, posterior). Overlap: raising of one fragment in relation to the other (which means shortening). Offset: rotation along the longitudinal axis of the bone. The lower fragment rotates externally or internally in relation to the upper fragment, causing the downstream limb segment to rotate in the same direction.

Displacement of articular fractures: Settling of bone tissue (and collapse of a corresponding articular surface). Separation of part of the articular epiphysis by a vertical or oblique line. These two "basic" types of displacement may be isolated or combined. In either case, they modify the joint profile. These different fracture structures and profiles were observed in the cliches presented to us by the patients.

11.5. Types of lesions

In ZE Kane's "therapeutic village", traumatic fractures were the most frequent lesions, due to the acute and noisy nature of the trauma, which led patients to consult a doctor most often immediately afterwards. Traumatic lesions could have a spontaneously favourable evolution, leading patients to believe, rightly or wrongly, in the therapist's effectiveness. These lesions varied greatly, particularly in cases where the diagnosis was obvious and the patient presented with X-rays, we noted articular fractures, extra-articular fractures, dislocations and sprains. As a result, in the course of his practice, the therapist was able to see all the disorders of the musculoskeletal system, from the simplest to the most serious.

11.5.1. The seat of traumatic injury

Traumatic injuries were mainly to the limbs, with a higher percentage to the lower limbs. In the course of our study, we found that injuries to the lower limbs mainly involved the leg and tibia, with accidental falls and carelessness on the public highway accounting for a large proportion of patients consulting traditherapeutes. Concerning laterality, the right side was the most affected, which corresponds to the general population, the majority of whom are right-handed in our country.

Table 1: Representation of fractures by lesion site

Nature of evil in Bulu	Nature of evil in French	Seat of lesion	men	women	children	total
Mvou'ou	fracture	Arm	01	01	01	03
Mvou'ou	fractures	collarbones	02	00	00	02
Mvou'ou	fracture	Tibia and perone	04	00	00	04
Mvou'ou	fractures	femurs	02	06	00	08
Mvou'ou	fractures	Column vertebral	01	00	01	01
Dou'ou	strains	ankle	01	01	00	02
Dou'ou	sprain	The thumb	01	00	00	01
Dou'ou minsis	dislocation	ankle	00	01	00	01
Dou'ou minsis	Knee	knee	00	01	00	01
Total						23

CONCLUSION

The occurrence of a fracture does not wait, it is generally an accidental case which, depending on the means available and the care infrastructures available, directs or guides the patient's choice of treatment. Some cases are referred to hospitals as soon as the trauma occurs, while others opt for traditional treatment in "therapeutic villages", as in the case of patients who come to ZE KANE for treatment of bone diseases.

CHAPTER III

TREATMENT OF BONE FRACTURES
IN THE ZE KANE THERAPEUTIC VILLAGE

INTRODUCTION

In his article "*La description en actes. Que decrit-on, comment, pour qui?*" Yannick Jaffre (2003:6) wrote: "*the activity of description is presented as consisting in establishing a direct relationship with the world. To describe is to tell things as they are, taking care not to 'add to them' with one's own ideas or feelings. Understood in this way, this activity contrasts with others that are more 'subjective', and supposedly more complex, such as imagining or interpreting*. In this chapter, we want to show how ZE KANE Samuel and his son MONAYONG Martin care for patients with bone disease who arrive at their bone disease unit, which is ZE KANE Samuel's "therapeutic village". To better support our description, it will be presented in different sequences. We will begin by characterising our study population, followed by the activities involved in the actual provision of care.

III. Characterisation of the study population and requirements of care staff.

In the "therapeutic village" of ZE KANE, two members of staff work in this traditional health structure: ZE KANE Samuel and his son MONAYONG Martin. The father and son work together on patients' cases. The father transmits his therapeutic knowledge to his son, who already works full time when he is on site. When the son is away, the father treats the patients.

III.1 Identification of the "therapeutic village" nursing staff
III.1.1. Therapist ZE KANE Samuel (Actor N°1).

Grandfather ZE KANE Samuel was born on 20 June 1930 in Nko'olong. Son of KANE MONAYONG andNYAGONE Ether, he was a Yedjok resident in his native village. After completing his secondary education at the Adventist College in Nanga-Eboko, ZE KANE Samuel trained as an accountant in Ebolowa. After obtaining his diploma, he began by working in shops, running his own small business, then went to work for the FAO in Kribi, leaving the FAO to set up his own business. He then went to work for SICK, and later became a guarantor at SCHEL KRIBI, where he worked as a guarantor manager. And when his father saw that he was already at the end of his life, he said to him: "*My son, I'm going to die soon, come and look after the village*". Fulfilling his father's wish, he gave up his job and lost all the money he had invested in the business. In 1960, ZE KANE Samuel moved to the village of Nko'olong and married his first wife, Ada Marie, with whom he had one child. Today, aged 94 and a widower, he devotes himself to passing on all his therapeutic knowledge to his son and to his Adventist religious activities in Nko'olong.

1.1.2. 2. The therapist MONAYONG Martin (Actors N°2)

MONAYONG Martin was born on: 20 June 1960 in Nko'olong. He is married and has several children. Son of ZE KANE Samuel and ADA Marie. After his secondary education, he went out to look for work. He started out as a temporary teacher at IRAD in Nko'olong, then was recruited as an auxiliary assistant teacher to work in the Extreme-Nord region. In 1985, he passed the competitive examination for assistant teachers. After his training, he first worked in Dschang, but after some administrative problems, he returned to the village. He was then re-recruited by HEVECAM.SA as Head Teacher on 18 March 1992, where he remained until 2020, when he retired and has now been working full-time as a bone disease therapist in Nko'olong for two years.

111.2. Patient presentations (Actors)

In our film production we have chosen a patient named EYOMAN Christiane. Born on 09/03/1976 in Kribi. Widow and mother of two children. After her secondary education she got married and trained as a hairdresser and beautician. In 2OO7 she lost her husband. She now works as a hairdresser in Kribi while running her small poultry farm in Bidou III. She found herself in Nko'olong at the ZE KANE "therapeutic village" following an accidental fall in which she suffered a traumatic shock. Christiane was chosen because her healing process was taking place while we were in the field collecting data.

For a holistic view of care practice in this "therapeutic village", and in order to contrast our data, a retrospective study over three consecutive months, from November 2021 to January 2022, enabled us to interview twenty-nine (29) other people, comprising eighteen (18) patients, six (06) guards, seven (07) elderly people and two (02) health care staff from the Adjap Yessok CMA.

The inclusion criteria were the choice of traditional treatment for trauma in the "therapeutic village" of ZE KANE, the patient's ethnicity, sex and age. The non-inclusion criteria were patients who had not received traditional treatment in the "therapeutic village" of ZE KANE, patients who had been treated outside the study period, and patients who had been treated in a hospital. Our sample consisted mainly of people with fractures aged from 04 to over 85 years, health care staff from the therapeutic village, health care staff from the Adjap CMA, sick nurses and elderly people, in order to understand the fundamental reasons for the choice of traditional fracture treatment and bone disease care practices in this therapeutic village.

111.3. The requirements of the therapeutic village

Patients who come to the therapists ZE Kane and his son, are subject to a certain number of rules and protocols throughout the course of treatment:

Depending on the patient's case or the site of the lesion, he or she will need a nurse. This person is responsible for assisting the patient in all his or her movements. This is to ensure that the patient does not move the fracture site too much, which could lead to complications.

Buying a massage pot. Each patient has their own massage pot to reduce the risk of transmitting infectious diseases.

Blades for incisions. Each patient is responsible for keeping these blades clean and protected throughout the treatment process.

The therapist's breakfast kit (a packet of sugar, a tin of liquid milk, a tin of matinal).

The "Toufa": this is a symbolic sum that the therapist asks patients to pay before going into the bush to look for medicines. This "Toufa" amounts to five thousand francs for ZE KANE and his son MONAYONG Martin.

Once everything is available, the therapist can begin the search for the medication.

111.4. THE ORIGIN OF KNOWLEDGE AND ELEMENTS OF CARE
III.4.1. Origin of knowledge

The treatment of trauma in Ze Kane's "therapeutic village" is a family heritage passed down from generation to generation from father to son. Kane Monayong, ZE Kane's father, passed on the therapeutic knowledge of trauma treatment to his son at the age of 10, and ZE Kane in turn initiated his son Monayong Martin at the age of 12, who also plans to pass on the therapeutic knowledge of trauma treatment to his children. Since passing on their knowledge of bone care, ZE Kane and his son have introduced new tools for treating trauma patients to keep up with the times. This is the case with the x-ray click, which in the past was not required of patients, but which is now an "obligatory" tool, required of patients before they can receive any treatment. This requirement for a click contributes to efficient practice. The site of the fracture is "almost" localised, and the therapist can then use his or her expertise to use strategies to immobilise the site of the lesion and begin treating the patient.

III.4.2. ELEMENTS OF CARE

In this section, we describe the composition of the remedy used in the therapeutic village, and the fracture immobilisation tools used by practitioners.

III.4.2.1. The "Ndoup

Ndoup" is the main name of the medicine used to treat trauma in ZE Kane's "therapeutic village". Ndoup" is a black powder made up of four elements. Each of these elements has a role to play in the treatment of patients suffering from trauma, and among them is one that our informants were kind enough to show us during the preparation: the "Ndik", the main element whose use is governed by the following protocol: The therapist looks for the "Ndik" (lianas) in the forest, cut into several small pieces, which he leaves in the attic to dry for an indefinite period of time, taking them from the attic each time he needs them to prepare the "Ndoup". The other three ingredients used in the preparation of the medicine are secrets shared only by the therapists. Once all the ingredients and products have been assembled, the therapist can prepare the medicine. Once the 'ndik' has dried thoroughly, the traditional practitioner takes the pieces and places them in the fire to obtain the embers, which are then removed and crushed to obtain a black powder. This powder is combined with three other elements to make up the remedy used in the therapeutic village of ZE Kane, a medicine known in the Bulu language as 'ndoup', which means powder.

Photo 4: the Ndoup

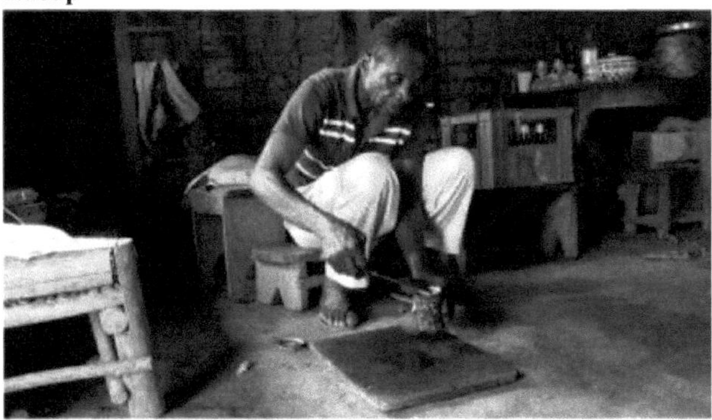

Source: *image du terrain photo Zongo Meric le 10/12/2021.Nko'olongPreparation du " ndoup ", " village therapeutique " Monayong fils de ZE Kane prépare le " ndoup " pour ses patients ;*

The "Ndoup" is the basis of all trauma treatment in ZE Kane's "therapeutic village", whatever the patient's case, the medicine used is the "Ndoup". The preparation of the "ndoup" (composition) depends on the patient's case, i.e. for a cranial trauma for example, the preparation of the medicine will be different from a fracture of the tibia, or a shock to the inside of the stomach (rib). The ingredients used to make up the remedy are the same, but in different doses, depending on the type of trauma or the patient's ailment. For example, the patient will be asked to take 'ndoup' for a trauma to the rib to drain the blood from inside the stomach. In the same way, the patient may be asked to do some head shots for a cranial trauma to limit memory loss, and also to make sure that he or she has a good memory.

1 to be applied to the site of traumatic lesion after incision in the majority of cases of fracture, sprain, dislocation, etc., of a limb of the body.

III.4.2.2. The preparation of "Obe Biang" (1'infusion of massage)

The infusion for the massage is made from the bark of trees known as "mindik" (lianas) and leaves. Once the ingredients have been collected, the therapist boils the mixture or asks the patient's carers to boil the massage pot. One to one and a half hours are needed to prepare the massage infusion. This infusion will be used throughout the patient's treatment. The use of the ingredients of the remedy is explained by our informant in the following terms:

Qmz : Why does Papa Moh use leaves for treatment ?

Rzk: I use the leaves in the treatment because you know that every remedy, every disease has its medicines and the medicines we use to treat us black people are these leaves from trees, herbs and tree bark.

Qmz: "Can you tell me how you prepare your remedy?"

Rzk: "But why not, I start by going into the bush to look for the leaves and barks that I've combined. I put them in the pot and boil them, and that's already the cure.

Qmz: "When you finish preparing this medicine, how do you use it?"

Rzk: "When you have an illness in the chest, when you have a trauma to the chest, then if I decide to incise the chest where you had the shock, then I also take the "ndoup" of the remedy that I use to give him to eat. He eats this powder that I put in his mouth like this. As soon as he finishes sucking, and it's already in his stomach, this product will work inside. If the blood wanted to coagulate in the chest, this blood would disintegrate, and as for what's in the stomach, this product finishes combining all this blood and finishes disintegrating this blood which ends up coming out. (Silence) ".

Qmz: "Thank you very much.

Rzk: "And it's also this same product which, if the trauma is in the head, as soon as you finish massaging the head, you finish cutting with the blade on the head, so you take this remedy and apply it to the head and I make another powder which doesn't sting, it's this powder that the patient sucks in like "nson" (tobacco), it's what goes to work on the head as far as the brain so that you don't have a brain disorder".

Photo 5: The massage pot

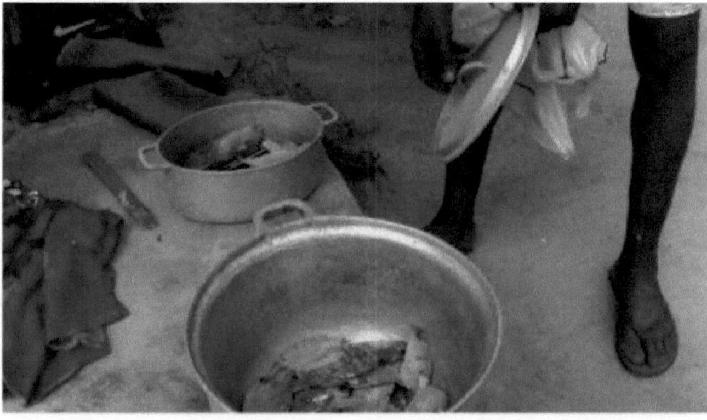

Source: *Image from the field. Photo Zongo Meric on 11/12/2021. Nko'olong: the "therapeutic*

village" massage infusion pot. Monayong prepares a massage infusion for two newly arrived patients.

As the treatment and care of the patient takes place on a daily basis, these infusion pots will be heated for a hot massage. This hot infusion decoagulates the blood at the site of the traumatic lesion and relaxes the veins that have received trauma.

III.4.3. Manufacture of immobilisation tools

In the ZE Kane therapeutic village, depending on the case of the patient presenting to the trauma care unit, the therapists use their ingenuity to immobilise the fracture and limit movement of the fracture site as much as possible. These include the manufacture of braces and cages.

111.4.3.1.   "The Akang

The "Akang" (cage) is a tool for immobilising the site of the injury. It is made from well-sized bamboo raffia and well-cut lianas that the therapist weaves to the size of the fracture site. It is used if the fracture is on a lower or upper limb. This is the case for fractures of the tibia, femur, arm or forearm. The role of the "Akang" is to keep the fracture immobile, as the patient in a fracture situation must not move very much for fear of aggravating the pain. This tool is the basis for all types of immobilisation in ZE Kane's 'therapeutic village'. Preparing the materials and making the "akang" can take from two to two and a half hours. The weaving of the cage obeys a certain number of indicators for evaluating the treatment process. Our informant told us:

QMZ: "How do you make a cage?

RZK: "You start by looking at the site of the fracture, then you take a piece of bamboo and clean it normally, then you cut the bamboo so that it extends a little beyond the two ends of the bone. Once you've finished cutting, you start weaving. You take the ropes, even the ropes from the trunks of plantain trees, which is what's preferable, so you take these ropes when they're dry and start weaving like the "nkonde".

But I've told you that when you weave you don't squeeze the ends of the cage together, you leave a gap where you'll know that the treatment is progressing normally."

And when the two ends of the cage do not stick together, this alerts the traditherapeute that the treatment is not progressing normally. The two ends of the cage must stick together to indicate that the fracture is progressing well.

Photo 6: Akang

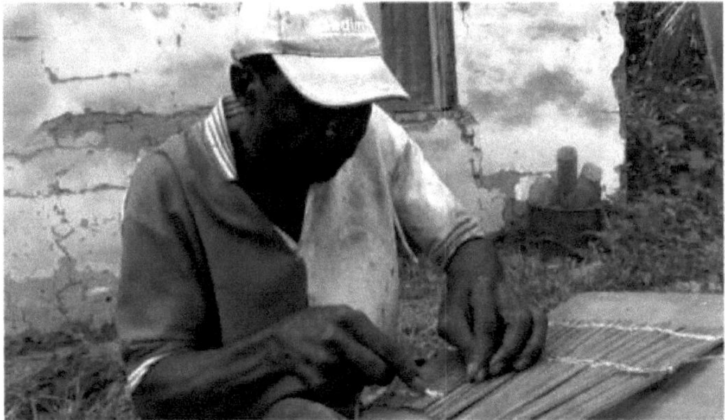

Source: *Image from the field. Photo Zongo Meric on 17/12/2021. Nko'olong: making the "akang", a fracture immobilisation tool in the "therapeutic village". Monayong makes the "akang" for a newly-arrived patient.*

The weaving of this immobilising tool has its origins in the daily life of the Bulu communities, who make cages because they began by sleeping on the "mineng" of the beds (the round wood) on which they used to sleep. And, after gathering them together, they then worked on the raffia, the bamboo raffia, making the stalls that were already there, the cocoa cages or the cages on which we sleep that we call "nkonde", so this "nkonde", The way they made it, that's also how they adopted it when a person suffered a trauma and fractured a bone, so that all the bones that had fractured and crumbled could be joined together to immobilise the fracture. To do this, when making the cage, the manufacturer has to make a cage that allows all the bones to be attached in a package that allows the bones to develop normally, so that they grow and stick together.

111.4.3.2. The boards

Therapists ZE KANE and his son MONAYONG use planks for certain fractures. These are small, well-sized pieces of counterplate, which help to immobilise the fracture.

Photo 7: Immobilisation boards

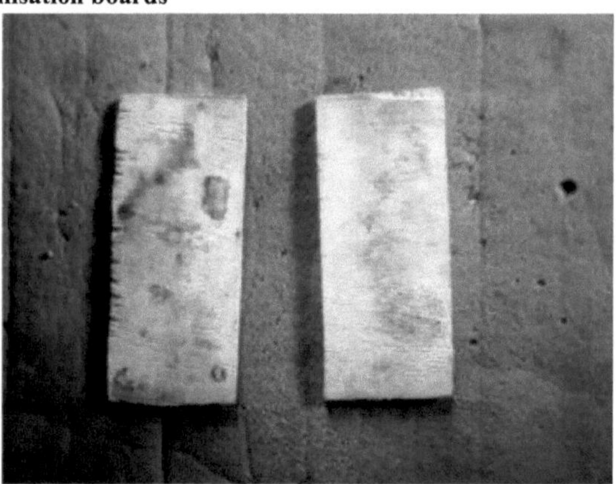

Source: *Image from the field. Photo Zongo Meric on 10/02/2022. Nko'olong: boards as a tool for immobilising fractures "therapeutic village".*

111.4.3.3. Chinese bamboo

Depending on the case, the therapists use strategies and imagination to immobilise the fracture and consolidate the bone. The Chinese bamboos are carved according to the site of the fracture. It could be a fracture of the tibia, arm or forearm. This tool is used to stabilise the fracture by bandaging it with fabric or tape.

Photo 8: Chinese bamboo

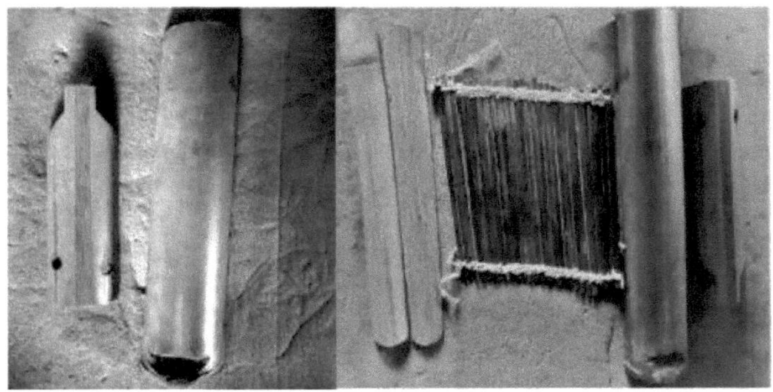

Source: *Image from the field. Photo Zongo Meric on 10/02/2022. Nko'olong: Chinese bamboo as a tool for immobilising fractures "therapeutic village".*

III.5. REDUCTION, MASSAGE AND SCARIFICATION

Fracture repair in ZE Kane's "therapeutic village" follows a protocol that ZE Kane's therapists and his son MONAYONG initiated a few years ago, namely: requiring an x-ray, massage, scarification and application of the drug "ndoup".

III.5.1 Therapeutic itinerary of patients and history of the click by the therapist

The ZE Kane therapeutic village is home to two types of patient, whose itinerary varies according to their illness and the treatment they receive. In fact, there are two types of patient: patients with 'papers' and 'undocumented' patients. According to tradi-therapist ZE Kane, 'paper' refers to a document issued by a public health worker to a patient at the end of a consultation. It may be a prescription, a consultation booklet describing the type of illness the patient is suffering from, apart from trauma, the results of a clinical examination or an X-ray image. The patient who has arrived presents himself or herself or the members of his or her party. If the patient has any documents to present, such as prescriptions or slides, he or she presents them to the therapist, who asks questions about the period when the trauma occurred. In general, it was found that patients arriving at the ZE Kane care unit follow three types of therapeutic itinerary for their pain: After a case has occurred, the first group of patients go directly to a hospital for treatment. If these patients are not satisfied with biomedicine, they may look for ways and means of using traditional medicine, in which case they may end up at ZE Kane for treatment.

The second group consists of patients who immediately go to the ZE Kane therapeutic village for treatment after a case has occurred. Depending on the patient's case, the tradi-therapist may ask for an X-ray before any intervention, or start the intervention by putting the patient under observation for a week. If there are no complications after observation, the patient continues to be treated until he is cured. At the end of the treatment (healing), the patient is asked to have an X-ray to check that the healing has been effective. If, on the other hand, the patient shows signs of a complication, he or she is immediately referred for an X-ray to determine the type and structure of the fracture, and the traditional therapist does not resume treating the patient until the type and structure of the trauma revealed by the X-ray has been confirmed.

Others come from other "therapeutic villages" where the treatment has not worked well. These patients are admitted on presentation of an X-ray with a medical image, and the traditional therapist begins treatment.

III.5.2. Patients without cliche

According to tradi-therapist ZE KANE, "paper" refers to a document issued by a public health worker to a patient at the end of a consultation. It may be a prescription, a consultation booklet describing the type of illness the patient is suffering from other than a fracture, the results of a clinical examination or an x-ray click for bone diseases. Patients from a variety of backgrounds arrive at the ZE KANE care unit following a traffic accident, an accidental fall, or carelessness on the public highway leading to a situation of shock, trauma or fracture. Some patients arrive at ZE Kane without being consulted by a doctor, nurse or healthcare staff when the physical shock or trauma occurs, due to a lack of financial resources, poor traffic flow and a lack of nearby healthcare facilities. They were admitted to the treatment unit and ZE Kane or his son MONAYONG Martin began treatment.

During our time in the field, we found that patients are referred immediately to the appropriate treatment unit, depending on their condition. If a patient's case is deemed manageable by the therapist, he or she is admitted without being referred to a hospital for an X-ray. If the therapist considers the case to be serious, the patient is referred to hospital for an X-ray. This was the case with patient EVE'E Jean Yves, who sprained his thumb during a fight, and whose therapists began treatment after he was brought to the treatment unit. And the case of patient EFFA Moise, the victim of a felling accident, whose case was deemed serious by therapist MONAYONG and who was referred to Ebome hospital (Kribi) for an X-ray. The X-ray revealed a double fracture (the tibia and the peroneum). On his return, he was admitted to the care unit to begin treatment. For others who presented without a cliche, therapist ZE KANE informed them that they would remain under "observation" for a week. If there was no change in the patient's condition, he would be referred to a hospital for an X-ray before continuing his treatment.

111.5.3. Patients with cliche

Generally speaking, when patients arrive at the ZE KANE care unit, they want them to present themselves with a "paper" (cliche) issued by health staff. This realisation came about when a patient came to the ZE KANE care unit some twenty years ago with an X-ray click showing a tibia full of fragmentary cracks. It was on the basis of this case that ZE KANE began asking patients to have an X-ray examination, so that he could see the site of the lesion more clearly and treat the patient more effectively. If the patient has a picture, he or she is admitted to the treatment unit. ZE KANE and his son MONAYONG admit the patient and begin treatment. They accept cliches that are no longer than three months old because, they say, the patient may have had another shock during this period, which could alter the structure of the fracture. The patient is therefore advised to have another X-ray of his or her injury if the period for which he or she is presenting has already exceeded three months. Because patients who arrive with a click may have other traumas after the X-ray examination, it is preferable for ZE KANE not to make a mistake in his analysis of the click by requiring the patient to feel the click.

III.5.4.1. The advantages of cliche

The treatment of fractures and bone diseases in the ZE KANE "therapeutic village" has led to a demand for an X-ray image of the patient's fracture. This allows therapists to benefit from the contribution of modern medicine in the care of patients suffering from trauma. The click allows the *"almost exact"* position of the fracture to be known, and limits the time taken to treat the patient, because when the therapist knows *"almost exactly"* the position of the fracture, it makes it easier for him or her to treat the patient.

1 operation. The cliche limits fracture complications. Many fractures are complicated because patients have not had an X-ray of their injury.

III.5.4.2. The disadvantages of the click

When radiologists are unable to reveal all the structural aspects of the fracture, it makes it difficult for the doctor or traditional therapist to make a clear diagnosis to the patient, which in the long term, if the anomaly is not detected quickly, can lead to complications and prolongation of the patient's treatment in the most serious cases.

III.5.5. Analysis of the click by the therapist

In ZE Kane's "therapeutic village", the medical imaging cliche has been introduced to the practice of treating bone diseases, to confirm or validate the diagnosis made by the therapist. It's a tool that's *"very, very useful, because the cliche shows you all the positions of the fracture, when the people who take the cliche have taken it properly, they've taken this fracture without hiding anything"*. In some cases, the image does not clearly show the site of the trauma. In these cases, it is necessary to use the skills of a bone therapist or to carry out a more in-depth analysis by means of a CT scan. As our informant explains:

QMZ: *"Can you tell us how you received patients before the cliche was introduced into practice?"*

RZK: *"If I talk about cliche, cliche has two things. The cliche doesn't bother me enough, because when the cliche arrives, some cliche like a Fang who was paying the.de kribi. He went to Ebolowa to get some money, so instead of going back to Kribi straight away, he first went to Edea, where he rolled over, so when they arrived with his cliche, he was first treated there in Edea. But when they came to show me his cliche, I told him that this cliche at the level of the anus, ga is going to bother you, this anus, the bone that is stretched out and he said to me "no, do you see when they made arrows, do you see an arrow there?" I told him that even as there is no arrow at this level, they didn't see it, they didn't see this part, they didn't examine this part properly. So this person did. He was already starting to show signs of healing, he was already getting up and going to sit on the veranda, but in the end, where I had said he would have a problem, this part had already started to hurt. He was the one who paid the inspectors and went to Ebolowa to collect their money. At that time Fam Joseph was a departmental inspector here in Kribi so I called Fam Joseph who took him to Kribi, he took this person to Kribi, (hospital) Kribi they said they could not. When they took him to Douala, where I showed, the slit that I showed, so when they did what they often do, um... I know they call it what? Er... The big X-ray... "*

QMZ: *"Scanner?*

RZK: *"Scanner, when they did the scan, then they discovered that the barrel he made three times, his kidneys were touched, it was already starting to swell and ga was already starting to rot that's why he died. Because it's over there in Douala. So if, what they did to Edea, if they saw this thing, they would treat it very well and when he arrived to be treated, he would perhaps be cured. So I know how to look at the picture, I know how to look at the picture very well, perhaps even surpassing those who do these things. Because I know the human body, I know the human body from the head down to the sole of the foot, I know because I studied it at school. I don't heal fractures by tattooing them and saying "no".*

Complications in patient care often arise when the structure of the patient's fracture is not properly determined by radiologists. It is therefore necessary for therapists to use their knowledge of the human body to provide the best possible care, or if necessary to request more in-depth examinations, such as a CT scan.

Photo 9: the click

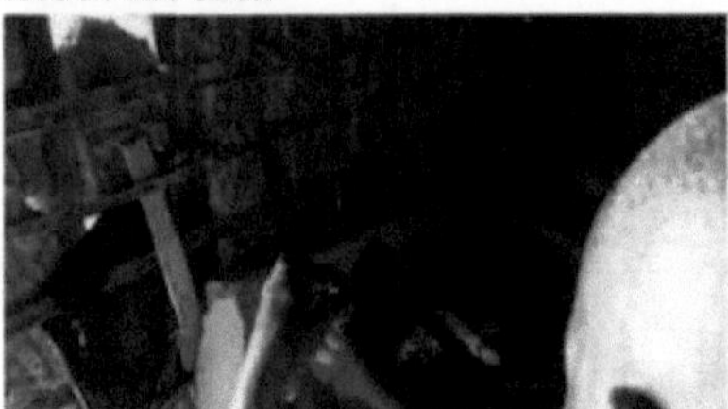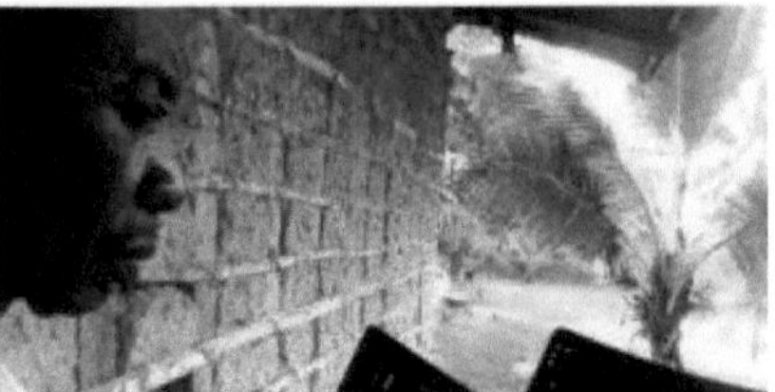

Source: *photo Meric ZONGO 24/12/2021. Nko'olong Analysis of a patient's X-ray image by ZE Kane Samuel and his son Monayong "therapeutic village".*

Some radiologists, when producing medical imaging images, fail to identify the site of the trauma by indicating it with arrows, which sometimes makes the work of traditional healers difficult and makes it difficult to treat patients. Traditional therapists therefore need to have a good knowledge of the human body if they are to treat patients more effectively and avoid the complications associated with misdiagnosing the condition. For the traditional therapist, the use of these two types of medicine provides added value in the care of patients in his or her unit.

III.6. Reduction

In simple terms, reduction can be seen as all the means and techniques used to treat the fracture with a view to returning the fractured bone to its normal state. According to the encyclopaedia, reduction is the first stage of treatment, the aim of which is to replace or return something (the fragments) to the normal axis of the fractured bone to ensure perfect repair. Some patients arrive immediately after their accidents at ZE Kane's "therapeutic village" for treatment. The first treatment carried out by the therapist is a reduction to reduce the pain that the patient is suffering. For the therapist, this means putting the bones and joints back in their proper place. In this respect, the therapist declares that :

QMZ: "Do you touch your patients when they arrive?"

RZK: "There are two types of patient. For some patients it's the day of their fracture (...) There's no other way if the patient arrives you have to do the treatment. Because if he arrives, if he's fractured today, and he's brought in, I have to finish putting the foot or arm back together when the bones have fractured, I finish putting them back together, I don't wait, I give him the treatment".

It's not good for the therapist if the patient arrives writhing in pain and doesn't return for treatment. The therapist will therefore immediately try to stabilise the patient so that the pain is reduced.

111.7. Massage

The massage is carried out by therapists using the infusion of bark and leaves that they look for in the forest when there is a case of fracture. The massage tool here is called "anyassa" (a pack of treatment leaves). Each patient has his own massage pot. To massage, the therapist first heats the infusion, then takes the anyassa, puts it in the water, removes it and starts to apply it to the area of pain. He massages by applying the "anyassa" from the top to the bottom of the fracture site, using a back and forth movement, which ensures that if it is a bone that is fractured, when the bone grows, it will not be a bump. This sliding movement of the "anyassa" ensures that the fracture site is *"protruding"* and well straightened, which is why

the therapist must apply the "anyassa" by pressing gently and do so with great care.
Photo 10: Massage

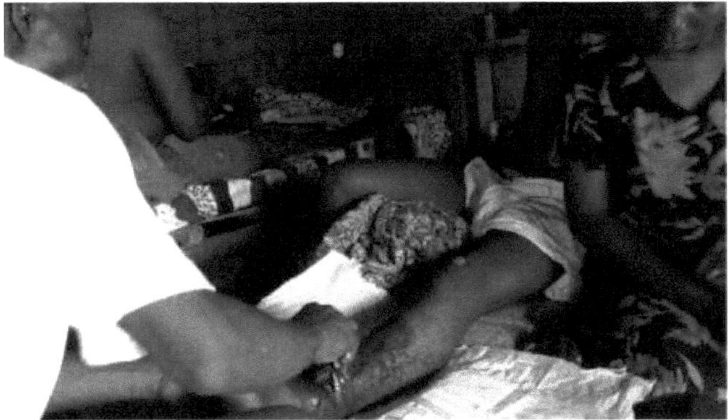

Source: *field photo Meric ZONGO, 13/01/2022, Nko'olong. Therapist Monayong massages a patient with a double tibia and peroneal fracture using a massage tool known as "anyassa", or "therapeutic village".*

For some bones, when they are not completely broken by massaging them with force, they can break completely. This hot infusion massage has the function of decoagulating the patient's blood at the site of the lesion, and also reduces the pain of the fracture. The massage helps to straighten the veins and improve blood circulation. The massage infusion is used throughout the treatment period. Each day of treatment, the pots are reheated without losing their potency, as our informant explains:

QMZ: *"How long do you use the infusion of barks and leaves?*

RZK: *"When I treat a fracture, using leaves and tree bark, you keep these things, these elements last a long time ga can do two to three months if the water is already finished, you can add because the remedy of leaves and bark does not permeate quickly ga has strength every time".*

The leaves and barks used by the therapist retain their potency because these elements are generally stored in very good conditions. The infusion is heated every day before the patient is treated.

111.8. Scarification

Scarification is a crucial stage in the treatment of fractures. Patients in pain are relieved by small incisions made by the therapist with a razor blade in the shape of a stick, which draws out the blood that could otherwise clot and cause the pain of the fracture.

QMZ: *"How does Papa Moh incise patients?"*

RZK: *"I then incise the people if I finish massaging, then I take the blade and I incise on the place that I finished massaging where there is the disease I incise there, and the blood comes out. When the blood has already finished coming out, then I take the "ndoup" which I apply even if the blood continues to remove this powder, without any problem the fact is that these wounds will already have regretted the power of the remedy."*

At that precise moment, while the therapist is making the incision, the patient is writhing in pain. And as he screams, he points to the place where he is in severe pain. In other words, you have to go through the pain to heal the pain.

Photo 11: Scarification

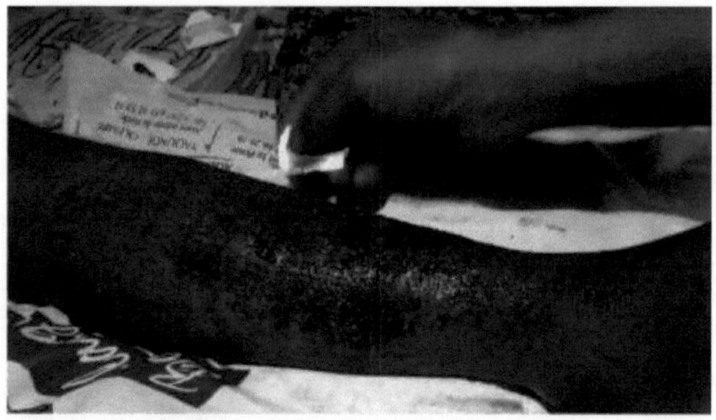

Source: *photo Meric ZONGO, 09/01/2022, Nko'olong. Scarification of a patient after a massage. "Therapeutic village*

For patients who do not show where they feel the most pain on the previous day, the next day, the night becomes difficult to bear because of the pain caused by *"bad blood"* that has clotted and does not allow good blood circulation.

111.9. APPLYING THE MEDICATION AND BANDAGING
III.9.1. Application of the drug

Ndoup" is a remedy used to treat fractures in ZE Kane's "therapeutic village". It's a black powder made from charred 'mindik' (liana) and other ingredients that are secrets shared only by the therapists. This powder has several functions in the treatment of a case. Ndoup" has several functions in the patient's body: Ndoup" ensures that if a patient's fracture is caused by fragmentary cracks in the bone that have spread throughout the body, *"Ndoup" brings these small pieces of bone back into place. Ndoup is an anti-tetanic, which is* why therapists use razor blades.

Photo 12: Application of Ndoup

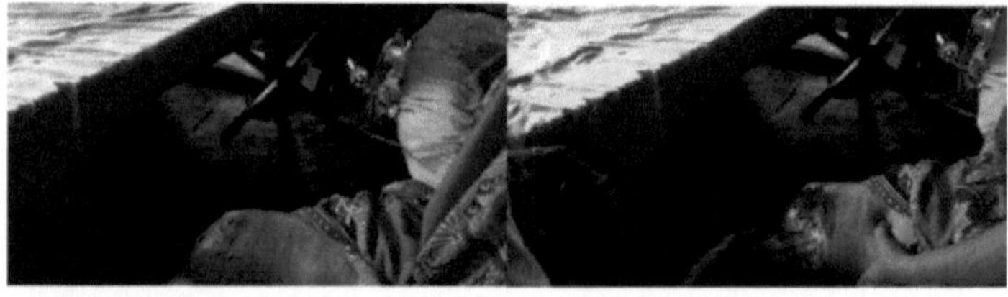

Source: *photo Meric ZONGO, 09/01/2022, Nko'olong. Application of the "ndoup" fracture remedy in the therapeutic village of ZE Kane. This remedy is applied after the patient has been scarified. "Therapeutic village*

We have also observed that 'ndoup' is not only applied to wounds, but can also be consumed by the patient or used to take 'ndoup' by inhaling it. This remedy can be used to relieve seizures in certain cases of head trauma. As our informant said:

QMZ: "When you finish preparing this medicine, how do you use it? Is it just for massage, or do you also drink it?"

RZK: "No, it's that when you have an illness in the chest, when you have chest trauma, then if I finish incising the chest or you've had the shock, then I also take the "ndoup" of the remedy that I use to give him to eat. He eats this powder that I put in his mouth like this. As soon as he finishes sucking, and it's already in his stomach, this product will work inside. If the blood wanted to coagulate in the chest, this blood would disintegrate, and as for what's in the stomach, this product finishes by combining all this blood and finishes by disintegrating this blood, which ends up coming out".

This is the same product that is used if the trauma is in the head, as soon as you finish massaging the head, you finish making the incision with the blade on the head, so you take this remedy and apply it to the head and the therapist makes another powder that doesn't sting. It's this powder that the patient takes from the head by sucking it in like tobacco, this is what goes to "*work*" on the head as far as the brain to limit brain disorders. After applying the ndoup, the patient will feel sharp pain for two to four minutes because the ingredients making up the ndoup sting, which prevents the "bad blood" from coagulating in the patient's body.

Ш.9.1.1. The drying time of the drug

The incisions made in the patients allow a lot of blood to flow out, so it takes a long time for the remedy applied to the patients to dry. This drying time can range from 15 to 20 minutes, depending on the amount of blood released by the incisions.

1.1.2.   2. The bandage

There are three stages to bandaging a fracture: the first bandage, the positioning of the cage and the second bandage.

1.1.2.1.   1. Why the first bandage?

The lesion is bandaged after the "ndoup" has been applied. In fact, after applying the remedy, it takes ten to fifteen minutes for the wounds to dry out with the remedy. If the wounds have finished drying, the therapist begins to bandage them by tying the bandage to the arm, foot or thigh. He starts by applying the first bandage. This bandage prevents the bamboo of the "akang" from touching the new wounds made after the incision. However, for certain indigent people, he sometimes ties up with pieces of cloth if the person does not have a velvet bandage.

1.1.2.2.   2. Positioning the "akang

The "akang" or fracture immobilisation cage is generally used if the patient has fractured the arm, the tibia or the peroneum, generally for long bones. This is when the therapist can position the "akang" on a patient. As the patient does not have to move enough, this cage allows the fractured bone to stick together so that it does not come loose or move. It immobilises and guards the bone so that it does not leave its seat where it fractured. It keeps the ends together until the bone has finished healing.

Photo 13: The akang

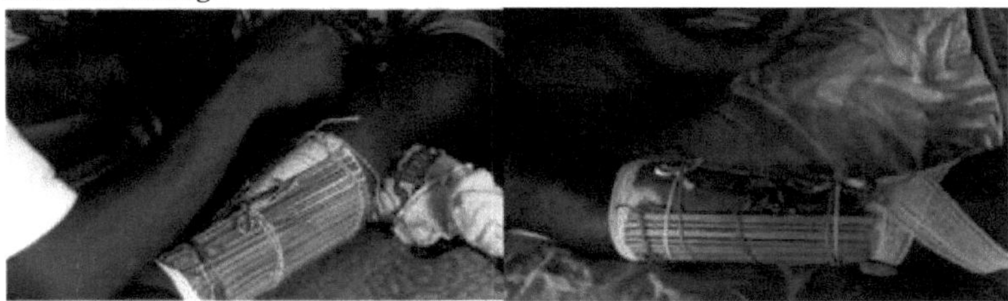

Source: *photo Meric ZONGO, 09/01/2022, Nko'olong. Positioning the "akang" after the first bandage. "Therapeutic village*

1.1.2.3.   3. Why a second bandage?

When the therapist has already finished tying the cage, then he takes a second strip. The first one is there to prevent the bamboo from touching the new wounds, so if he finishes tying up the cage, he takes another strip and puts it on the cage so that it looks good. Because "*the symmetry of the eyes is good*". And as the treatment is carried out every day, these same exercises are repeated every day of treatment.

However, once the patient has begun the healing process, he or she will start the treatment after two days, until leaving the ZE Kane therapeutic village.

Photo 14: *The second bandage*

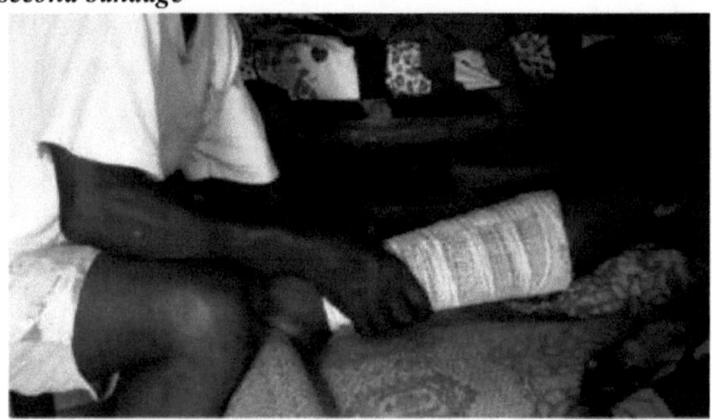

Source: *photo Meric ZONGO. From 09/01/2022 The Monayong therapist applying the second bandage after positioning the "akang". The "therapeutic village".*

The patient will wear this cage for as long as his body accepts, until his body heals and when the therapist knows that the fracture has already healed, and also knows that the bone has already adhered, it is at this point that he lets the cage be attached or removed, as the cage cannot be removed at any time during the treatment period.

Patients' bones stick together depending on their age. In fact, the therapist knows that a patient's bone has already bonded when the patient is a child, a young child when he or she has already had four weeks of treatment, for children the bones bond after one to two weeks and then the third and fourth weeks are for solidification.

And for people who are young men and women, when it has already been three weeks, particularly in the case of new fractures, it takes three weeks for the bone to set and by four weeks, it has already set well. However, in the case of old fractures, treatment starts as early as a month and a half, or two months, to allow the bone to solidify.

111.10.   Monitoring patients

Once a patient has been admitted to ZE Kane's "therapeutic village", they are obliged to follow all the therapist's recommendations to ensure they receive the best possible care. This supervision of patients includes certain prohibitions that patients are obliged to respect throughout the period of their treatment. As the treatment is carried out every day, the therapist also assesses the progress of the treatment. Usually two weeks into the treatment, the therapist can already determine whether or not the treatment is progressing normally. The patient must refrain from greeting (shaking hands with) all visitors during the entire treatment period, to avoid transmitting bad spirits, as the therapist takes to be the case:

QMZ: "Why do you forbid your patients to shake hands with their visitors?
RMM: "Do you think all the people who come here come with a good spirit?"

Visitors are not allowed to sit on their beds,

For the patient's own safety, it is forbidden to drink alcohol,

A ban on sexual relations with a partner throughout the treatment period.

Also, in certain cases, if the therapist considers the case to be serious, he himself may abstain from sexual intercourse:

QMZ: "Why abstain from sex?"

RZK" When you say that you treat people you must have abstinence so when you treat people, you don't follow women even if you have your wife you don't touch her just as the patient also must not "go out" so when you are clean like ga, the treatment works well but if you see a treatment with complications, now ga it's already as if like ga, difficult, difficult two months, three months without cure you will know that there is a difficulty if you want we also show you that like ga... you yourself will also betray".

When some of these prohibitions are not respected by the patient, the treatment time is prolonged, complications can be observed, and in some cases even manifest themselves in the massage pot. And the therapist knows at that moment that the patient has not complied with the instructions.

Traditional practitioners monitor their patients on a daily basis, as the treatment is carried out every day. To encourage consolidation, they ask or advise patients to eat a diet rich in calcium, such as fruit, sardine oil, etc. Consolidation is achieved after a specific period, which is set at two weeks for children, three to four weeks for young people and five to six weeks for adults. When the patient reaches six to seven weeks, he or she is taken to a rehabilitation phase - walking, for example, is sometimes authorised with a cane as soon as the pain disappears, or the therapist may ask the patient to carry out an activity if it involves an upper limb. This phase occurs two to three weeks before the bone solidifies.

## 111.11.	REEDUCATION

Following a traumatic shock and the fragmentation of the healing process, appropriate rehabilitation is essential. The aim of this is to restore full function to the joint, strengthen the musculature which has generally atrophied during long-term immobilisation, and prevent recurrence or (Visio callus). In fact, ZE KANE and his son MONAYONG Martin adopt several strategies to help the joints regain their functional mobility.

Ш.11.1. Upper limbs

Once the bone in the arm, forearm or wrist has solidified perfectly, the ZE KANE tradi-therapeute puts the patient through a motor activity such as holding objects. For women, he may ask them to go fishing to see if the arm can already perform motor activities. In the case of men, he asks them to clear a yard, for example. If the patient manages to do this without any complications or difficulties, he or she is ready to leave the "therapeutic village". On this subject, our informant states that :

QMZ: "I'd like to talk about how you teach your patients to do things again if it's the foot, how they should walk, how does that often happen?

RZK: "I tell him... I tell him to walk maybe as far as the church when he's already walking like that I tell him to go as far as the entrance to Jerusalem city. Then I ask him to go to the other side of the village to the entrance to IRAD. When he manages to do that, that's it. Because when he comes back without being tired, and he himself feels that he has the strength, I tell him that he can already leave".

QMZ: "How long does it take for a person to learn to walk again?"

RZK: "It also depends on the strength of the patient. Because some people are weak. There

comes a time when they can already walk, but if they're weak, there's no fixed time for that. If I see that I've asked someone to walk and they can't, I ask them to wait a little longer. I ask him to wait another week and then I ask him to walk".

Some patients undergo three to four weeks of rehabilitation once their bones have healed. Once the automatisms have been acquired and the patient feels able to do exercises, he or she may wish to be released.

III.11.2. Lower limbs

Similarly, in the case of a fractured lower limb (e.g. the tibia, femur or ankle), once it has fully healed, the therapist begins by lifting the patient to a standing position for at least seven days with a cane. The procedure consists solely of standing without walking, as immobilisation causes patients to lose their balance, so they must regain their balance before walking again. Once the patient has regained their balance after seven days, they can begin to take their first steps in the room. The therapist also has distances for the patient's walking exercise. He can ask the patient to start with a distance of 100 metres with a crutch, depending on the patient's mobility and resistance, and the therapist increases the distances. The patient will walk for one to two weeks with the crutches, then the therapist will remove the crutches from the patient, repeating the walking exercise until the patient feels able and asking the therapist if he or she is ready to go. This walking exercise without crutches can take from two to three weeks, depending on the patient's adaptation.

III.12. ABANDA'A: the shielding ritual

The "abanda'a" or the armouring of a patient against fracture is only done if the patient asks to be armoured. So, after the patient has fully recovered and is ready to leave if he asks to be armoured, the therapist asks him to bring chicken, a litre bottle of palm oil, all the condiments and a diet of walled plantar as a complement to the meal.

When everything is ready, the therapist slaughters the chicken, the patient, or the patient who has been kept sick, de-feathers it and the therapist returns to skin the chicken.

In ZE Kane's "therapeutic village", the patient is asked to provide four elements of armour to prevent fractures: a chicken, a litre of palm oil, all the condiments needed for cooking and a diet of ripe plantain.

III.12.1. Preparation of chicken and plantain

The chicken is first prepared in a pot with all the condiments needed for cooking with red oil. The plantain is also prepared in a pot. When the chicken is already cooked and tender, the chicken and plantain are mixed in the same pot. At the end of the cooking time, the therapist can come and perform his ritual by introducing the remedy into the pot. The patient, or his nurse, can take charge of cooking the meal. After cooking, the therapist puts the remedy into the pot and then begins to share the meal with those present for the occasion.

III.12.2. The meal

All the food is placed on a banana plantain leaf *and* after placing all the food on the leaf, the patient is served, usually two pieces of chicken, followed by this sentence:

"All this is your food if you want it, you can give it to people".

Showing the food placed on the sheet. During the meal, all those taking the meal are advised not to break the chicken bones, so they are asked to watch each other and the therapist himself. After the meal, all the chicken bones are collected and placed on the "witness" sheet.

Photo 15: Shoring meal

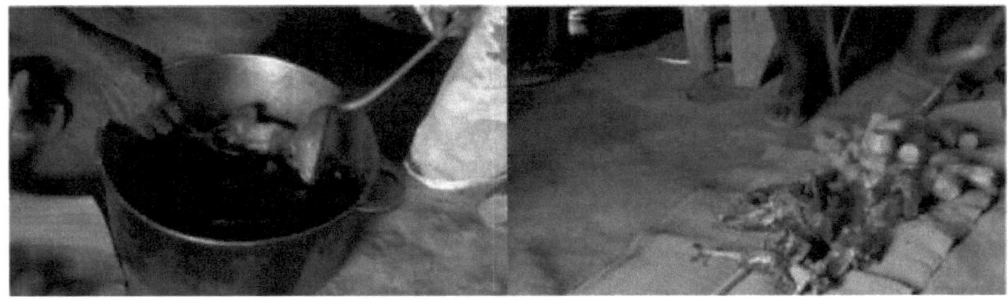

The therapist comes back to check that all the bones haven't been broken, then packs up all the bones and goes off to '*throw*' them in the bush, where even stray dogs won't be able to destroy them.

This armouring ritual is designed to ensure that even if the person who has been armoured finds himself in a situation where he could break, this will not happen. On this subject, our informant states that :

QMZ: "Why armour a patient against fracture?

RZK: "We armour the patient at the fracture centre so that (...) The armouring is so that you don't fall ill again. When we say shielding, we mean that we close you up so that you don't get sick again. If you fall, you won't break again. So that you don't break again (silence) Yes, that's why you do the shielding".

QMZ: "All the patients who have already come to you for treatment and whom you have blinded, they can no longer (...) If they have broken, they can no longer break?

RZK: " il ne vapas se casser. The one to whom I've given armour won't break.

QMZ: "How did Dad Moh make this happen?"

RZK: "How do you do it? When you treat a patient for an illness, you treat him so that he doesn't get sick again. Treating an illness (fracture) is part of the treatment, and shielding the patient is also part of the treatment. The disease is attenuated, this illness, the armouring is done to attenuate the disease even if you've reached the point where you can break, you're not going to break".

Patients who have received anti-fracture armour can no longer be *"subject to fracture under any circumstances"*. The patient is asked not to provoke circumstances that could lead to a fracture. After the meal, the ex-patient of the ZE Kane "therapeutic village" can go home to his family and say goodbye to his doctors and his "colleagues" in the disease.

Caring for a fractured patient treated in the therapeutic village of ZE Kane is therefore not limited to medical treatment (ndoup, Obee Biang), but also reveals a *"mystico-religious"* dimension embodied by the traditional therapists of the therapeutic village of ZE Kane. By treating the suffering body, the therapist also seeks to prevent future harm.

CONCLUSION

Traditional fracture treatment has developed considerably over the last ten years. Traditional medicine, which remains a cultural heritage, is deeply rooted in the therapeutic choices of African populations, particularly in Cameroon. To provide better care for their patients, traditional therapists use strategies that are adapted to the different cases they deal with, and they also introduce modern medical tools for effective care. To this treatment of physical and psychological trauma are added rituals of protection not only against the forces of nature, but also against mystical forces.

CHAPTER IV

PERCEPTIONS, REPRESENTATIONS AND INTERACTION IN THE THERAPEUTIC VILLAGE

INTRODUCTION

In this chapter, we aim to analyse and interpret patients' therapeutic choices in the ZE Kane 'therapeutic village' by answering the question: What are the reasons for patients' referral to therapeutic villages? To do this, we will first look at perceptions and representations, and then at the interactions between the tools, the patients' therapeutic itinerary and the practice of care in this traditional health structure specialising in bone repair, which will enable us to gain a better understanding of the care practices used for bone disease.

IV.1. PERCEPTIONS AND REPRESENTATIONS

Our analysis of trauma care practice in the therapeutic village of ZE Kane is based on the perceptions and representations that therapists and patients have of the two types of medicine in general and trauma care in particular. For the traditional therapist, traditional medicine is a tool for *'relieving the spirits'* of patients. The strength of his practice lies in the divine principle that has given him the gift of healing. Even in the case of a *'mystical'* fracture that is *difficult to heal*, the practitioner knows that, by divine force, he will be able to get to the end of the case. Our informant reaffirms this conviction in the following terms:

"(...) I am not a man of evil spirits, I heal all cases of fracture by the power of God. If you arrive, even if they've done something to you, even if they haven't done anything to you, if you arrive, I pray to my God. Because what I'm doing is praying to God to give me the strength to look after her child. Because his child has had a problem, may he give me the strength to look after him, even if it's the kind of broken bones I've just finished treating".

The practice of trauma care in ZE Kane's "therapeutic village" is a family heritage passed down from generation to generation from father to son. It follows a therapeutic protocol initiated by the therapists in order to perpetuate the practice and care of patients suffering from physical and psychological trauma. Once the patient has been presented to the care unit, the treatment is based on the following points: In the event of a new fracture, if the patient presents immediately after the accident, the traditional therapist may, if necessary, perform a reduction, which consists of putting the fractured bones back into place.

In addition, to provide more appropriate alternative care, if a patient's case is deemed serious, he or she is referred to a modern health facility for a medical imaging examination to identify the structure or type of fracture in the patient. This biomedical analysis tool, which gives the structure of the fracture, has been introduced into traditional trauma care practice to enable the traditional healers of the "therapeutic village" to treat trauma patients more effectively. Patients therefore prefer to come to ZE Kane's 'therapeutic village' because they know that their illness is the work of the *'enemy'* and that the therapist who is the guarantor of traditional therapist knowledge can find a solution to their health problem.

For all of our informants, traditional medicine is a traditional heritage to be preserved, protected and conserved with great delicacy, because therapists are precious depositaries of therapeutic knowledge in communities *"do we have anyone else?"* having an inestimable value, they have a role to play within the whole population. There is no difficulty of access, because everything is there and patients find it interesting that care is given to the patient from the moment he or she enters until the moment he or she leaves - these repositories of traditional knowledge are in our communities. The patient is immediately admitted to the care unit, with or without money, and the therapist is with the patient every day. This daily assistance to the patient enables the patient himself to see how his case is progressing. The reasons for traditional treatment vary from case to case and from patient to patient. Asked about patients' perceptions of traditional medicine, one of our informants said that :

Qmz: "What do you think of traditional medicine?

Rec : Traditional medicine even as many still neglect qa, but I assure you that these are the herbs that God created for us, he gave us the power to use them we must no longer neglect qa because traditional medicine many still neglect qa many who have not yet had cases like this because at first I myself neglected but today, I can already see how traditional medicine is helping our country and the whole world, even herbs and barks, everything that God created is useful to us. Traditional medicine is doing wonders all over the world at the moment. I'm not trying to contradict modern medicine, but the two must be taken at the same value, because I've told you about my foot, the state of my foot, and how much it cost to treat it here, how much it cost at less than forty thousand euros, and whether it was in hospital, I'm not saying that they do anything wrong or that they don't provide treatment over there, but I'm talking about what happens in traditional medicine.

The local people, who have difficulty accessing hospitals and whose access to the therapeutic villages is facilitated by their proximity and the "*appreciable*" quality of the care they receive, see the practice of traditional medicine, in view of its contribution to patient care, as a health tool that should be considered to be of equal value to modern medicine. For them, the two forms of medicine must work together, as the WHO wishes. In this regard, Tchoumi Tchouli E 2020 added that "*Our study does not claim to resolve all the controversies surrounding the analysis of health problems, in particular that of the chi-skymi-therapists in our study area*" (pp 100).

Combining the two types of medicine will enable patients to be treated more effectively for many illnesses. If it is accepted that the purpose of caring for individuals is to relieve suffering, its function is also not only to heal the suffering body but also the patient's mind and sometimes to prevent (circumstances). This is why we hope to see a slice of collaboration between practitioners, from the traditional to the modern and from the modern to the traditional and vice versa, and that the patient is at the centre of health policy aimed at his well-being.

Similarly, the cost of treating the patient is a determining factor in the choice and therapeutic orientation of patients towards therapeutic villages. The image that some people initially had of traditional medicine is tending to disappear. Traditional treatment was once seen as something to be laughed at, as a lack of resources, as destitute - in short, as someone who did not want to be cured, to be healthy, to be physically and spiritually well.

But today, through the various achievements of traditional medicine, the therapeutic itineraries of patients today make it possible to understand that many patients in search of health have recourse to traditional medicine, which they recognise as having a significant contribution to make in the treatment of trauma, and they call for collaboration between the two types of medicine. Traditional medicine and the holders of this traditional therapeutic knowledge are therefore not people to be ignored. Traditional medicine needs a great deal of encouragement from the government and administrative authorities to encourage research, because traditional healers also need the support of the authorities and the government. Supporting them will enable even more research to be carried out, to develop and improve the ways in which patients are cared for and looked after in therapeutic villages, in order to provide tools and solutions on how to treat trauma in the plural.

IV.2 Patient reception facilities

QMZ: "Where did you get the idea of creating a place to keep the sick?"

RZK: "You know that when you have a visitor, you have to give him a place to stay. You have to give them a bed and a place to stay. And when he says he's being looked after, he's already your child, he's already your stranger, he's already your person.) The disease doesn't catch just one person and the disease doesn't avoid anyone, especially fractures, so I've seen that if I already have the remedy to treat fractures, I have to have a house (hospital) in this house, I make beds if there are resources, I put mattresses on the beds so that a patient who arrives can make his own bed. And I have to put in several beds because as the patients arrive, none of them have to lie on the floor. The patient must sleep on the bed, each patient must have his own bed".

It was this expression of love for one's neighbour that inspired ZE Kane to set up a facility specialising in the treatment of bone diseases, a traditional health institution that has now been in operation for over fifty years. This facility, which is able to admit patients from a variety of backgrounds, enables them to keep all their treatment appointments. Respect for human life and the conditions provided for its "*children*" have made the therapeutic village of ZE Kane a benchmark facility for the care of trauma patients, as one of our informants, a patient at the therapeutic village of ZE Kane, testifies.

QMZ: "Does Grand Patric have anything else to add regarding the facility, the nursing staff and the other patients?"

REN: Yes I'm going to add something by saying really, I'm first going to thank all this entourage because, it's not even what I thought I'd find, but it's the opposite of things. Because at first I said to myself that I've never lived with this ethnic group, so that would be, ... Given that I do not have a nurse and my girlfriend is not there she works, she can not leave work for here. But the opposite of everything, the old, everyone, I am more than Kribi, I am very, very well received, and ga gives me really too, too much courage and really I thank the whole village in a word. What I didn't think I'd find here is the opposite of everything, it's really going to be very serious in my mind even when I leave here, I won't forget, I won't forget this family. Yes, they'll be like a second family to me - we've even started, the familiarity's already there. Given that..., I'd say the young doctor's wife is a cousin of mine from the same village as Papa Batanga. All right, all right".

QMZ: "The family gets together?

REN: "Yes, well, the family is back together, so I'm very, very, very satisfied, very, very satisfied, thank you very much".

It is this spirit of conviviality that drives the ZE Kane care structure. Here, despite the modest conditions in which patients are treated, they find themselves part of the human condition. Relationships are established between traditional therapists and patients, and between patients themselves. ZE Kane's therapeutic village is intended not only as a structure for caring for patients who have suffered trauma, but also as a social structure where the well-being of the patient and the individual is a major concern for the therapists. ZE Kane and his son MONAYONG Martin.

IV.3. Medicines

The main remedy is an infusion of barks and leaves for massage, together with "ndoup", which is applied after incising the fracture site. The "ndoup" remedy is the basis of all treatment for trauma. Depending on the case presented to the treatment unit, the therapist composes the "ndoup" that will be used to treat the patient's ailment. The final medication, if the patient so wishes, is anti-fracture armour, which reduces the risk of fracture for a patient who has been armoured. After the patient has been cured, he or she may, if he or she so wishes, ask for an anti-fracture brace. Counter fracture. Shielding is carried out if the patient so wishes after his or her recovery. It reduces the risk of fractures in all circumstances.

QMZ: Why do we armour a patient against fracture?

RZK: We armour the patient against fracture so that (.) The armouring is so that you don't fall ill again. When we say shielding, we mean that we close you up so that you don't get sick again. If you fall, you won't break again. So that you don't break again (silence) Yes, that's why you do the armouring.

QMZ: "All the patients who have already come to you for treatment and whom you have blinded can no longer... If he's broken, he can't break again?"

RZK: "He's not going to break. The one I've finished armouring isn't going to break.

QMZ: "How is Dad Moh doing?"

RZK: "How do you do it? When you treat a patient for an illness, you treat them so that they don't fall ill again.

The treatment of an illness is a part and the armouring is also a part so that he doesn't fall ill again (silence). We attenuate the illness, this illness, the armouring is done to attenuate the illness even if you've reached the point where you can break, you're not going to break".

IV.4. Therapists' perception of traditional medicine

For therapists, traditional medicine requires a relationship of "ndi" (trust and or faith) to be established between therapist and patient if treatment is to be effective and efficient. This 'ndi' relationship enables the treatment to progress more effectively. The patient is asked to have firm faith in the practice of his or her therapist.

IV.5. The two types of medicine

Fracture repair or trauma management in the Cameroonian context is a multi-faceted form of care. Many traditional structures are already starting to integrate biomedical analysis tools into their patient care. This is a requirement of Cameroonian government policy, and a collective awareness on the part of traditional therapists to improve patient care. This is the case for ZE Kane's "therapeutic village", which has introduced the requirement for patients suffering from trauma to have an X-ray film with a medical image. Acknowledging the authority of Cameroon's Ministry of Public Health, and fearing the problems associated with the risk of complications arising from treatment, the traditional therapists at the ZE Kane therapeutic village ask their patients if they have seen the hospital that issues them a 'paper'.

This document may indicate any illness suffered by the patient and help the tradi-- therapeute to better understand the patient's case. In some cases of trauma care, certain 'doctors' who recognise the 'merits' of traditional medicine in Cameroon refer patients to therapeutic villages for trauma care, and vice versa. Similarly, in some cases, when the traditional healer finds that the patient who initially arrived with a trauma has a pathology (contagious disease) other than the trauma, they call on the staff of the district medical centre, which acts as the district health inspector, to come and observe the patient. However, the deontology and ethics of the medical profession oblige hospital staff to refer patients by category.

In Cameroon, traditional healers accept hospital staff into their care structures in order to provide relief to patients (as in the ZE Kane therapeutic village). *"We go to them for advice"*, says a nurse. Although these hospital staff know that certain pathologies and traumas can be treated using traditional medicine, they still refuse to treat patients in the plural, i.e. in a way that allows them to be treated using both modern and traditional medicine, depending on the case and the illness from which the patient is suffering. Because, they say, they respect the ethics and deontology of their profession. The raison d'être of medicine is to relieve the suffering of individuals in society. While it is true that Africans recognise that there is such a thing as evil, just as there is such a thing as good, no society can evolve without the means to ward off misfortune or consolidate the good. This is why the traditional therapists at the ZE Kane therapeutic village do not deviate from this logic when treating their patients. It's true that there are cases of natural trauma in certain situations. However, humanity is convinced that there are also cases of trauma that are not natural but are planned or provoked. In fact, this is the main reason why traditional therapists are consulted in most cases of trauma.

In the treatment of illnesses in general, and in the therapeutic villages in particular, traditional practitioners are convinced that some cases of illness are 'launched' or caused by enemies, sorcerers lurking in the shadows, and that their role is therefore to *relieve the spirits* of these patients, who appear not to know the origin, or at best the source, of their ailments. Some patients therefore see the consequences of an invisible hand in their situation. It is because of this observation of a gloomy and mysterious world that a good number of patients in trauma situations seek solutions to relieve their ills from traditional therapists. These socio-cultural elements are researched and put in place by the proponents of traditional therapeutic knowledge through mechanisms that enable them to propose a solution to different cultural problems. This is what justifies the fact that in the treatment of a patient who has suffered trauma in the therapeutic village of ZE, Kane, the patient can, at the end of his or her treatment, if he or she so wishes, request armouring against fractures.

In the therapeutic village of ZE Kane, several tools are used to treat patients. In addition to the "akang", the "ndoup" and the splints, the village's traditional therapists have introduced the use of medical imaging to improve patient care. Patients are asked to take x-rays with a medical image, depending on the type of trauma they are suffering. This combination of practices contributes to faster patient recovery at lower cost. The cliche: a biomedical tool, the medical imaging x-ray cliche enables therapists to :

Identify the site or position of the fracture,

Identify the type or structure of the fracture,

The click shows all the positions of the fracture, and when radiologists take the click, and they have taken it correctly, the click helps in the care of bone diseases. However, it is important to note that it is necessary for the tradi- therapeute to master the practice of his work, to know the human body and to be gifted with imagination in order to take better care of patients' cases and the need for collaboration between hospitals and the "therapeutic village". Acknowledging the importance of collaboration with hospitals in the care of patients suffering from trauma, our informant put it this way:

QMZ: Thank you very much. Patients who arrive without a cliche how do you go about treating them?"

RZK: "You know that's an old job that people have always done, so I often tell them that (...), I tell such cases that I'm going to put you under observation here for a week, I'll treat you for a week if I see that there's no change, then I'll send him to hospital because hospital is very, very useful for him to do the X-ray. Because X-rays are very, very useful.

Once this tool has been analysed, therapists can begin treating the patient. To limit the risk of infection and complications, the patient needs to be monitored every day until he or she is completely healed. In addition to the need for a cliche to treat a patient's trauma, several other biomedical specialists come to the ZE Kane therapeutic village to treat patients with other types of illness. Proof that the ZE Kane structure has the patient's health at heart.

IV.6. INTERACTIONS IN THE THERAPEUTIC VILLAGE.

IV.6.1. Patients' lives

The patients, who come from different backgrounds, are called upon to stay and live together in the space offered to them by the therapist. Like any social space, relationships and interactions between individuals give rise to agreements and disagreements. The therapists, anticipating the conflicts that can arise in this space, give a line of conduct to all the patients who arrive in this care structure. Former patients pass on the guidelines directly to new patients, which helps to rebuild relationships. The patients in ZE Kane's "therapeutic village" live like a family with the same father and mother, and the circumstances that bring them together ensure that they live together, eat together, pray together - in short, that mutual aid prevails in this new socialisation space. Individuals from different ethnic groups come together in a new space and acquire new ways of living and sharing. In this respect, one of our informants revealed that :

QMZ: Do patients sometimes argue?

RZK: Well, yes, there are often arguments between patients.

But I've been told by the authorities that if there's a patient looking for trouble, I've got to get them to leave, because if the blood starts flowing, I'll be the first person to stop it, so I don't just accept trouble. Anyone who wants to make trouble I chase away.

In the event of a conflict, the therapist is the first to look for ways and means of resolving the dispute between his patients, because he considers them all to be his "*children*" and there is no question of his children being seen to tear each other apart. If there is a dispute between the patients, he sits them down and hears them, and the guilty party is blamed, with a ban on repeating the offence or risk being thrown out of the treatment. He reaffirms it in these terms:

QMZ: What can cause problems between patients? RZK: What can cause problems between patients is this: it's obvious that wherever people live, there are those who are genuine and those who counterfeit. So if a patient goes to trade on another patient somewhere, and when the latter is made aware of it, they start quarrels. Some people take out loans and don't want to pay back what they've borrowed. These things cause problems.

QMZ: "And how are these conflicts settled?"

RZK: "When there's a conflict between patients, I ask them what's going on. If they finish telling me what's going on, I tell the one who's wrong not to do it again, you're the one who's wrong, don't do it again, it causes arguments with the others, don't come here to cause problems and if it continues I'll kick you out.

At the end of a dispute, the patients are heard and the therapist looks for ways to resolve the conflict. If the protagonists do not want to listen to reason, the therapist may go so far as to expel the patient who has caused the conflict and the latter leaves the treatment. These cases are extremely rare, as the therapist favours dialogue between patients and mutual support.

IV.6.2. Patient/therapist interactions

Whatever the circumstances of life, when two, three, four, five or six individuals find themselves in the same place in the same circumstances, there can be problems. That's why ZE Kane, anticipating the derives that can occur in his structure, has initiated a line of conduct that all his patients are required to respect.

The instructions come from the district's administrative and health authorities, i.e. if there is a patient there looking for problems, that patient should be chased away and made to leave, because if there is a problem, the therapist will be the first person to be arrested, so this information is given to any new patient who arrives. Anyone who wants to cause problems is chased out of the 'therapeutic village'. And if a patient is suspected of having a contagious

69

disease, the therapist is asked to call the doctors, who come from time to time to check on the state of the facility and the health of the patients. To this end, the patients live in perfect harmony, helping each other, as one of our informants put it:

QMZ: "We're going to try to talk about your interactions with other patients, how do you live in this common room?"

REN: "In our room, because when I arrived I found some elders who directly gave me a line to drive, so since I've been here, we're like a family of 05, 6, 7 people, same father, same mother, we live together, we say hello, we have breakfast together, we eat lunch together, we have evenings together, we say prayers together, it's not individual, it's like a .... so in our room there's no exchange of words, we're like the children of a mother and a father, everything's really quiet".

QMZ: "So since your arrival you haven't had any crowded warm-ups with other patients?"

REN: "No, quite the opposite, quite the opposite, it's jokes, it's fun until 1am, it's comments about everything and nothing, it's like being in a house with mum and dad's children, so there's no arguing, no bad words, no, everything's rosy, everything's rosy".

The relationship between therapists and patients in the ZE Kane therapeutic village is one of conviviality, love, sharing and mutual respect. These are the values that govern the daily lives of everyone in the ZE Kane therapeutic village. And this is justified by the fact that many patients, after completing their treatment, express the wish to return and spend a few days here. What's more, they express the feeling that they have very good memories of their time spent in the therapeutic village of ZE Kane. Many of them also found a lover or a girlfriend here. Staying in the same place brings people closer together, and from time to time they form relationships, both friendships and romantic ones.

IV.7. Patients' therapeutic itineraries

When people feel ill, they need relief wherever they come from. In the case of bone fractures in our country, the situation is becoming increasingly difficult, as the country does not have enough orthopaedic specialists or bone surgeons, and treatment is becoming more and more expensive. In view of all this, individuals suffering from fractures are going to multiply the ways and means of seeking treatment for their case. In this case, we have identified five different types of therapeutic itinerary for patients:

Patients initially go to hospitals after their accident. If they are not satisfied, they move on to "therapeutic villages".

For others, after their accident, they go to "therapeutic villages". If they don't find a cure, they can look for other "therapeutic villages" like ZE Kane's structure.

For others, they arrive directly in ZE Kane's "therapeutic village". If the patient's case is deemed manageable by the therapists, treatment begins immediately. If they consider the case to be serious, they refer the patient for an X-ray and the patient returns for treatment.

Similarly, some people go through two or three hospitals before going to a "therapeutic village". One of our informants described his itinerary in the following terms:

QMZ: "Where did you go after your accident?

REN :After my accident, I started at Ebome hospital, where I spent about a week. There was no intensive care, there was nothing to evacuate me, I was evacuated immediately to the regional hospital in Edea, where I had a meeting with the Director of the hospital, Gustave TCHAGADIGUI, who is a bone specialist, I had a double fracture of the clavicle plus a dislocation of the left shoulder, so to make matters worse, the clavicle was even operated on, but the shoulder was not put back in its place, and that's where everything went wrong, with the certainty that when I came out of the operation on 14 July 2019, I'd have my arm back in December. Well, that wasn't the case, it was just in December that I found another opportunity, an opening that we were advised to go to an orthopaedic centre in Bepanda Boulangerie la paix where I was admitted and the doctor was also hopeful ha but, where we spent almost a year ten days ga didn't give that I made the remark I freed myself alone ga wasn't worth it.

It is necessary to release the places and to go to seek elsewhere done of the, I returned to the village in Kribi of course to spend practically one whole year without care, And then one day at the landing stage at home, given that the general management of the landing stage had given me a small Hall collection post, the director, Mr Nana Tabet Anicet, a Bamileke, told me Mr NGANDO, you were a brave fisherman here, given that you are handicapped at the moment, but at least with one hand you can manage, we give you the tickets and that's it, it's in the "done" tickets that I meet a girl, a young girl who asks me questions about how it is... I didn't want to at first, I was a bit tired of answering people's questions, of telling them a bit about my physical position, so the girl insisted because she wanted me to buy the fish from her, she was a friend, not a girlfriend after all, a friend, she insisted, insisted, then we moved on to the next stage, I told her, she said, well, we're going to go and do..,

Get yourself some money and we'll go and have a look around Nko'olong, there's a dad who's a healer, a bone specialist, and then we made an appointment and we went round, the old man examined me and gave me the details of what I needed to bring, so I respected that and I came back and we took the interview and the next day on 19 September, October 2021. From the 20th, the arrival was on the 19th, he started work on the 20th, so I'm a month and a half down the line. I'm confident, and you know, when a patient arrives at the hospital, whether it's with the "Ngueng- ngang" or at the hospital, he's always firmly convinced that he's going to get well again, so we're hopeful that one way or another he's going to be fine.

The quest for care means that patients have to move back and forth, depending on the case and the resources available, between modern health structures and traditional care structures. For the patient, the expected outcome of this to-ing and fro-ing is a cure. Different itineraries were observed among patients in the ZE Kane therapeutic village. Many of our informants chose different itineraries after their trauma.

IV.8. Auscultation of patients

Our informant tells us that patients used to be examined by hand. The therapist used his hand to feel the position of the bones, with the experience he had acquired, and one patient came in with a picture, which made him aware of the delicacy of the cases that could present themselves to him. The patient in question came in with a picture that showed cracks in the patient's tibia, like a bottle with cracks in it, and he was afraid that some cases were fractures, when they can be stopped with force, perhaps they are cracks and you end up with the whole foot crumbling (shattering).

Since then, in order to improve the effectiveness of his care, the therapist has introduced the requirement for patients to have an X-ray film. Nowadays, the vast majority of patients arriving at the ZE Kane health centre are asked to present themselves with an X-ray film, a tool that helps to improve **patient** care. In view of the results, the messages are being disseminated and passed on to people in fracture situations, and people are flocking to this therapeutic village. By integrating biomedical analysis tools into patient care in this way, traditional medical practices are being modernised, adapted and improved to provide better patient care.

IV.9. Care billing

Treatment for fractures in the ZE Kane therapeutic village is almost free. In fact, all the people we spoke to were satisfied with the way the therapist treated them. At the outset, the patient is asked for a pot for his massage tea, packets of blades for the incisions made during his treatment, a packet of sugar, a tin of milk, a tin of morning tea for the therapist's breakfast and a modest sum of five thousand francs for the search for medicines in the bush, and the therapist can begin his treatment whatever the case. At the end of the patient's treatment, the price of the treatment is negotiated at the patient's discretion. As our informant put it

QMZ: "How much does it cost to care for a patient in your clinic? RZK: "The patients who come to me, because we receive... I can tell you that we don't have a fixed price because the patients, and the plethora of patients who arrive here from over there, you know which one? When they finally get better... The patient you have faith in is the one who stays here, all those who come for treatment and leave don't trust them. Because as soon as the latter sees that he's already cured, even if you see him coming when he tells you he's going off to get some money, he leaves with no return. And I can't complain to the person. So what happens is that if the patient arrives, I ask him to buy his massage pot because patients don't mix remedies. You have your remedy because the blood is bad at this time there are diseases like AIDS and others. You buy the pot, your pack of blades is yours to keep if the blade doesn't cut any more, you take a new one, you give it to me and as soon as I've finished making the incisions, I give you the blade back. I also tell the patient that when they come in for treatment here, this is the ligot catcher. After buying your massage pot, you give me a box of matinal, a packet of sugar and a tin of milk, and when I go to collect the medicine, you give me five thousand francs, so even if you leave, if I finish treating you without any problems, I've had my share. And if you have a good heart, you finish the treatment, you ask me how much you have to pay me and I ask you how much you can pay yourself? If you tell me how much you can pay, you give me that amount and I take it. And if you say how much you can pay and you don't give it and you leave, there's no problem because I treat patients more to help their spirits."

QMZ: "So there's no amount you can charge for a patient with a fractured foot?"

RZK: "I can't lie about there being a fixed amount, because patients make up their minds as they go along. One patient might give me twenty thousand, another thirty thousand, another fifty thousand. But things are going to grow, because when I started I wasn't even taking five francs just because life has become difficult for everyone - is a kilo of rice still the same price as last time? So... We're also in a situation where if something happens it's often said that (proverb) maybe something bad can happen you see, when the authority comes to arrest you you have to know what you've done then, a sum you can tell a patient. Many of the people I treat I ask them to leave when I see that they can't pay for something, that they have nothing, I ask them to leave. In several cases I finish treating them and I ask them to leave, I don't ask you for anything, and also my people, those I know who are my relatives or foreigners who are not my relatives, if they tell me they have nothing I say they should leave.

This magnanimity is one of the reasons why the "therapeutic village" of ZE Kane is so popular. That's why it's rare for a case of fracture that occurs in this locality to be treated in a hospital elsewhere, but whatever the case, the first port of call is the "therapeutic village" of ZE Kane.

CONCLUSION

In short, the aim of this study was to describe the perceptions, representations and interactions observed in the therapeutic village of ZE Kane, by answering the question: What are the reasons for patients' referral to therapeutic villages? There are several reasons why patients choose traditional medicine for the management and treatment of bone fractures. The cost of treatment is almost free, the experiences of patients, the feeling of always being with family, the feeling of ineffectiveness of modern medicine through the different therapeutic itineraries, the time taken for treatment - in short, there are many reasons why patients choose traditional medicine for the care of patients who have suffered trauma.

GENERAL CONCLUSION

Humankind has always sought and found ways and means of curing illnesses that threaten its existence. Thus, in all parts of the world, at the same time as striving to adapt to different environments, man has been able to find and develop knowledge and practices to preserve his existence through products of natural, mineral, animal or plant origin (Tchoumi, 2021). This knowledge and practice, which we refer to as pharmacopeia and traditional medicine, is passed on and enriched from generation to generation, and is gradually structured and codified. This work is part of this process, which aims to present the contribution of traditional practice in the treatment of bone diseases. We have attempted to approach the problem from the angle of patient care in a therapeutic village. The phenomenon we have tried to explain is that which is enshrined in the concept of the 'central core', i.e. care practices. To explain this phenomenon, which is more than a result or indicator, it is a factor in explaining patients' therapeutic choices. We drew on the theories of social representations (Moscovici 1961) and on observational cinema through the concept of the 'participatory camera'. Overall, our aim was to answer the research question: **Why this desire to go to a therapeutic village for treatment of fractures?**

The aim of this research was to **highlight the contribution of traditional practices in the treatment of bone diseases in general and in the therapeutic village of ZE Kane in particular.** This led us to identify three specific objectives: to identify the mode of care and describe the socio-professional characteristics of patients who turn to the therapeutic villages in the event of a bone disease; to describe the care practices for bone diseases in a therapeutic village; and to describe the care practices for bone diseases in a therapeutic village.

therapeutic villages and, finally, to understand the rationale for referring patients to therapeutic villages. To achieve the objective of this research, specific steps were taken from the research protocol onwards.

The first part is designed to lay the theoretical and conceptual foundations without which this work would be devoid of all substance and meaning.

A second stage was devoted to operationalising our hypotheses and analysing the data collected in the field through interviews and observation.

The results obtained make it possible to establish the following causal links: The method of care and the social status of patients suffering from bone disease explain their use of therapeutic villages. Therapeutic care for patients suffering from bone disease follows a protocol established by therapists. Patients are referred to therapeutic villages for economic reasons and a sense of symbolic efficacy.

Research contribution

The aim of all research work is to make a significant contribution to a given problem, in order to advance science. The scope of this research is twofold: scientific and practical.

In scientific terms, this research will provide anthropology of health and research into traditional medicine with knowledge of endogenous knowledge, methods and practices for treating bone diseases in particular (fractures, sprains and dislocations).

From an applied point of view, this research is a tool that can be used to support decisions by the bodies responsible for health (WHO, Minsante), MINAC and UNESCO, to have a tool for decision-making with regard to the treatment of a certain type of bone disease, the conservation of therapeutic practices and the enhancement of endogenous knowledge and know-how.

The limits of research

In conclusion, at the time of writing, it should be noted that the objective of our study has been achieved. However, even if the objective of this research has been achieved, it is still true that, like any human work, it can be improved. The main limitation of our research work relates to the size of our research sample.

A look ahead.

As this research project draws to a close, we can look forward to a number of avenues for future work.

At the end of this research, it appears that, beyond the limits of the research, the objective of our research work has been achieved. An understanding, explanation and analysis of the reasons behind the use of therapeutic villages and care practices for bone diseases has been established. The contributions of this research have been presented, and the significance of this study in the context of Cameroon, and even the countries of the Congo Basin in general, should not be overlooked. It is therefore incumbent on researchers to take advantage of this work in future research in order to develop a genuine literature on traditional medicine in general and on bone disease care practices in therapeutic villages in particular.

BIBLIOGRAPHY

Marc-Eric Gruenais, 2002 " La professionnalisation des " neo-tradipraticiens " d'Afrique centrale " in Sante publique et Sciences Sociales N°8&9 Juin.

M. E. Gruenais, D. Mayala, "How can we get rid of the "symbolic effectiveness" of traditional medicine?"

Marc-Eric Gruenais 1991, "Towards a new traditional medicine in Africa: the example of the Congo. " Sans la priere, sans la danse, les potions peuvent-elles etre efficaces ? " " In la Revu du Praticien. Medecine generale, tome5 N°114.

Eliwo Mandjale Akoto, Paulette Beat Songue, Samson Lamlenn, Jacques Pokam wadja Kemajou et Marc-Eric, 2001 " Infirmiers prives, tradipraticiens, accoucheuses traditionnelles a la campagne et a la ville " in Bulletin de 1 APA D ; un systeme de sante en mutation : le cas du Cameroun.

Marc-Eric Gruenais, Laurent Vidal, 1994. "Medecins, Malades et Structures Sanitaires : Temoignages de praticiens a Abidjan et Brazzaville" in ORSTOM, Departement Sante UR, Societes, populations, sante 213, rue La Fayette 75480 Paris Cedex 10.

Annie. Walter. 1982 " Ethnomedecine et Anthropologie medicale. Bilan et perspectives" in cah, O.R.S.T.O.M. Ser, Ssci Hum. Vol XVIII. N°4 pp 405-414.

Fainzang. S, 2000 " la maladie, un objet pour l'anthropologie sociale " in Ethnologie Comparees Universite de Montpellier 3. France.

Fainzang. S, 1999, " L'Anthropologie medicale dans les societes occidentales ". In sciences sociales et sante, John Libbey. Pp 5-28

Olivier de Sardan. J.P, 2006 " Anthropologie de la Sante " In le dictionnaire des sciences humaines. S. Mesure & P. Savidan (eds). PUF. Paris. Pp 1039-1041

Reveyrand.O, 1983 " Etiologie et perspective de la maladie dans les societes modernes et traditionnelles ", Premier Colloque National d'Anthropologie Medicale. Paris.

Dozon. J.P, Sindzingre.N, 1990 " Le pluralisme therapeutique et medecine traditionnelle en Afrique contemporaine ", Fond documentaire ORSTOM N°30 Gando. A, 2006 Politique Nationale de Medecine Traditionnelle.

Auge. M, 1986 " L'Anthropologie de la maladie ", In l'homme, pp 81-90.

Niete Municipal Development Plan 2013

National Health Development Plan 2016

Mbonji Edjenguele, 2009 Sante, maladies et medecine africaine, plaidoyer pour l'autre tradipratique, Les Presses Universitaire de Yaounde.

Tchoumi Tchouli Elisabeth, 2020 Approche socio-anthropologique du recours au massage traditionnel lors des fractures humaines par la population de Ngaoundere 1er et 2eme memoire de master recherche Universite de Ngaoundere.

FILMOGRAPHY

Canal + Studio 2022, "Baby-Boom

Jean Rouch " l'initiation a la danse des possedes " (initiation to the dance of the possessed)

Pierre Tizi Lankissa 2020 "Scrap metal is our future

Ghislaine Magouo Tainon 2020 "Cabaret de Djebba

APPENDICES

Appendix 1: Attestation of Research

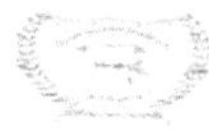

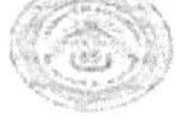

REPUBLIQUE DU CAMEROUN
PAIX-TRAVAIL-PATRIE
REPUBLIC OF CAMEROON
PEACE-WORK-FATHERLAND

UNIVERSITE DE NGAOUNDERE

THE UNIVERSITY OF NGAOUNDERE

FACULTE DES ARTS, LETTRES ET SCIENCES HUMAINES

Tél : (237)222254018/222264037

FACULTY OF ARTS, LETTERS AND SOCIAL SCIENCES

N° 0341/24 /UN/D-FALSH/CD-SOCIO-ANTHRO

Le Vice-Doyen chargé de la Recherche et de la Coopération

The Vice-Dean in charge of the Research and Cooperation

Ngaoundéré le 3 0 JUL 2021

ATTESTATION DE RECHERCHE

Le Vice-Doyen chargé de la Recherche et de la Coopération de la Faculté des Arts, Lettres et Sciences Humaines de l'Université de Ngaoundéré atteste que l'étudiant **ZONGO MERIC**, né le 28/11/1994 à Adjap, est inscrit en Master II recherche, au titre de l'année académique 2020-2021, dans la filière Sociologie, option : anthropologie visuelle suivant la décision N°2021/060/UN/R/SG/DAAC/D-FALSH/VDS du 05 mars 2021, sous le matricule 19B877LF. Il effectue, à cet effet, un travail de recherche sur le thème : « *Patrimonialisation des savoirs thérapeutiques traditionnels : les soins des fractures dans le village thérapeutique de Ze Kane Samuel à Niété* ».

Nous le recommandons auprès des institutions, organismes et personnes ressources susceptibles de lui fournir des informations nécessaires à la réalisation de son étude.

En foi de quoi, la présente Attestation lui est délivrée pour servir et valoir ce que droit

LE VICE-DOYEN

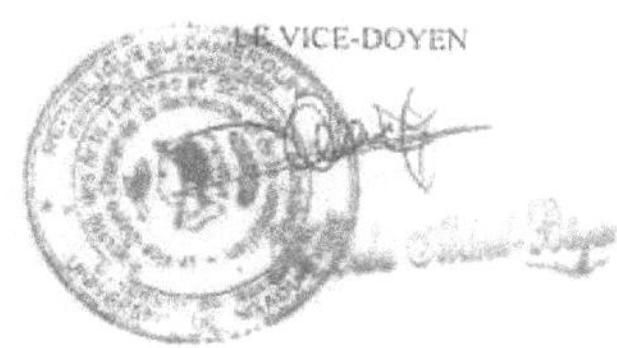

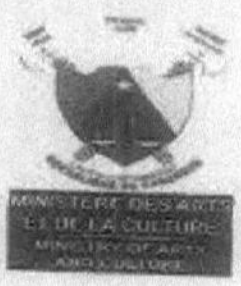

REPUBLIQUE DU CAMEROUN
Paix – Travail – Patrie

MINISTERE DES ARTS ET DE LA CULTURE

DELEGATON REGIONALE DU SUD

DELEGATION DEPARTEMENTALE DE L'OCEAN

B.P : 605 Kribi   Tel : 699244329
mbengvictor@yahoo.fr

REPUBLIC OF CAMEROON
Peace – Work – Fatherland

MINISTRY OF ARTS AND CULTURE

SOUTH REGIONAL DELEGATION

OCEAN DIVISIONAL DELEGATION

P.O.Box : 605 Kribi Tel : 699244329

Kribi, le 1 8 NOV 2021

AUTORISATION DE PRISES DE VUES CINÊMATOGRAPHIQUES
(PERMIT TO FILM)

VU LE DÉCRET N° 90/1462 DU 09 NOVEMBRE 1990, fixant les conditions et les modalités d'obtention des autorisations d'exercice de l'activité cinématographique.
In accordance with decree n° 90/1462 of 9th November 1990 to lay down the conditions and procedure for obtaining authorization to carry out cinematographic activity

AUTORISATION N° 14 /APV/RS/DDAC-O
Permit N°

VALABLE DU : 25 octobre au 31 décembre 2021
Valid till

EST ACCORDEE A : ZONGO Méric titulaire de la CNI n° 1158467709 du 26
Is given to :   avril 2012

QUALITE : Etudiant
Profession

ADRESSE : Ngaoundéré-Cameroun Tél : 655 091 765
Address

POUR EFFECTUER DES PRISES DE VUES CINEMATOGRAPHIQUES
To take film Picture

DANS LES LOCALITES CI-APRES : Village thérapeutique de ZE KANE Samuel

TITRE : Pratiques des soins des maladies des os à Niété.
Titre

RESUME : L'observation de la pratique des soins thérapeutiques et impressions auprès de patients.

FORMAT : Appareils photo, caméscope, téléphones.

EQUIPE DE TOURNAGE : ZONGO Méric

N.B. :
* La Délégation Départementale des arts et de la culture décline toute responsabilité en cas de modification, aux risques et dépens du réalisateur, du contenu du film après l'obtention de la présente autorisation.
* L'utilisation d'un drone requiert un accord de l'Autorité Aéronautique.
* « Aucune œuvre cinématographique, quels qu'en soient le genre et le format, ne peut être mise en circulation au Cameroun en vue de sa représentation en séance publique, à des fins commerciales, éducatives ou culturelles, si elle n'a pas obtenu le visa réglementaire délivré par le Ministère chargé de la cinématographie ». (Cf. article 18, al.1 du décret n° 90-1462 du 09 novembre 1990 fixant les conditions et les modalités d'obtention des autorisations d'exercice de l'activité cinématographique).

Le Délégué Départemental

PLEG

Appendix 3: Research Authorisation

REGION DU SUD

REPUBLIQUE DU CAMEROUN

Paix – Travail – Patrie

DEPARTEMENT DE L'OCEAN

ARRONDISSEMENT DE NIETE

SOUS-PREFECTURE D'ADJAP

BUREAU DES AFFAIRES ADMINISTRATIVES

JURIDIQUES ET POLITIQUES

LE SOUS-PREFET

A

MONSIEUR ZONGO MERIC

Etudiant à l'université de Ngaoundéré.

Ref : V/L en date du 17/11/2021

N° 005/L/L11-01-1/BAAJP

<u>Objet</u> : A/S demande d'autorisation
de recherche

Monsieur,

Accusant réception de votre lettre visée en référence dont l'objet est repris en marge.

J'ai l'honneur de marquer mon accord pour le compte de vos travaux de recherche dans mon ressort de commandement, portant sur le thème : « LE VILLAGE THERAPEUTIQUE DE ZE KANE SAMUEL PRATIQUES DE SOIN DES MALADIES DES OS A NIETE. »

A cet effet, vous voudrez bien prendre préalablement attache avec le Chef Traditionnel de 3ème degré Nko'olong abritant le site ciblé qui vous assurera les facilitations nécessaires.

Veuillez agréer, Monsieur, l'expression de ma parfaite considération.

<u>Copies</u> :

- Préfet/Océkbi : « ATCR »
- Chef trad. Nko'olong » p. info et dispositions utiles à prendre »

Adjap, le 1 0 DEC 2021

Le Sous-Préfet Par Délégation,
L'Adjoint

Barnabé Ndzama
Secrétaire d'Administration

Appendix 4: List of informants

Survey identification sheet

№	People surveyed	Gender	Age	Village	Ethnic group	Religion	Occupation	Level of study	Marital status	Type of fracture	Date of interview
01	ZE KANE Samuel	M	94	NKO'OLONG	BULU	ADVENTISTE	therapist	5th	VEUF	Therapeutic village	27/11/2021
02	MONAYONG MARTIN	M	60	NKO'OLONG	BULU	ADVENTISTE	therapist	2ndC	Marie	Therapeutic village	12/12/2021
03	ZE OKOTO Emilienne MAKON	F		ADJAP NKONTOCK	BULU	EPC	MENAGERE		MARIE	Femur fracture right	08/01/2022
04	CHARLES MEVA'A	M	23		BASSA	CATHOLIC	STUDENT	Tie	Single	Double fracture of the tibia, left peroneum	17/12/2021
05	SAMUEL	M	40	ADJAP	BULU	CBC	PLANTER	3rd	Single	Dislocation of the hip	31/12/2021
06	CHARLIE MENGUE CECILE NLATE	F	53	KRIBI	MABEA		Menagere		Single	Femur fracture right	18/11/2020
07	FELIX	M	38	ZINGUI	BULU	EPC	GENDARME	TThe	Single	Femur fracture left	25/11/2020
08	MBO'O ARNAUD	M	28	EBOLOWA	BULU	EPC	Student	TThe	Single	Fracture of the vertebrate column	22/11/2020
09	EYOMANE CHRISTIANE DESIRE	F	47	BIDOU II	BULU	New Church	Hairdresser	ER	Widow	Clearance and fractured tibia	13/01/2022
10	Mbo MARIE	F	68	Akok	BULU	EPC	Menagere		Widow	Older people	17/01/2022
11	SHEY VINCENT	M	62	TANKENG	WIBOM	Catholic	Mechanic	Cepe	Marie	Fracture	26/01/2022

№	People surveyed	Gender	Age	Village	Ethnic group	Religion	Occupation	Level of study	Marital status	Type of fracture	Date of interview
12	KABEYENE PHILOMENE	F	85	EDOUDOUMA	BULU	Adventist	menagere		Widow	Tibia/Peroneum Older people	14/01/2022
13	ATYAM MARIE CLAIRE	F	38	Nko'olong	Bulu	Catholic	Menagere	CEPE	Single	T radipraticienne	15/12/2021
14	EVE'E IEAN YVES	M	62	Nko'olong	Buhl	EPC	Contract	CEPE	Mariee	Sprain	10/01/2022
15	OKOTO OKOTO IULIEN	M	40	Nko'olong	BULU	EPCO	Agent de l Etat	CEPE	Marie	Notable/ Fracture of the tibia (left)	22/01/2022
16	NGOULA	M	32	BIVOUBA	BASSA	Catholic	Tracker	CM1	Single		28/01/2022
17	DAVID EVINA KENAN	M	4	Nko'olong	BULU	EPC	Student			Sick call Fractured arm (right)	02/02/2022

No	Name	Sex	Age	Place	Ethnicity	Religion	Profession	Education	Marital status	Diagnosis	Date
18	MAKON BORIS	M	27	NKONTOCK	BASSA	Catholic	Debrouillard	3rd	Single	Sick leave	28/12/2021
19	MINKO AMELIE	F	54	AFAN6OVENG	BULU	Catholic	Menagere	^eme	Single	Sick watch	15/02/2022
20	EYENGA MARIETTE	F	74	AKOMI	BULU	Catholic	Menagere	CEPE	Mariee	Femur fracture (left)	15/12/2021
21	NZIE LUC FERRAN	M	27	MEYO	FANG	Adventist	Debrouillard	CEPE	Single	Fracture of the clavicle (right)	29/12/2021
22	EKOUBE NGANDO PATRIC	M	37	MBOUA-MANGA	BATANGA	EPC	Pilot of tug	CEPE	Single	Fracture of the clavicle and dislocation of the shoulder (left)	29/12/2021
23	MINKOUA NESTOR	M	25	NLENDI	FANG	EPC	STUDENT	^eme	Single	Double fracture of the femur (left)	20/11/2020
24	EDJIDJI BERTINE MARIE-NOELLE	F	40	EDOUDOUMA	BULU	EPCO	COMMISSIONER OF PHARMACIE		Mariee	Sanle staff	09/02/2022
25	MEYE RAYMOND	M		ADJAP	BULU	EPC	NURSE		Marie	Sanle staff	09/02/2022
26	MIMPOUGA	F	56	NTSINDA	MAKA	EPC	Menagere	6th	Mariee	Hip	02/02/2022
27	EKOTO CLAIRE LYDIE MBOM MBOM JOSEPH	M		Y embong	Bulu	EPC	Debrouillard		Celibalaire	dislocation Sick watch	18/02/2022
28	OLOUN ESTHER	F	92	Zoe-tele	Esse	EPC	Menagere		Widow	Hip dislocation	18/02/2022
29	MFOUM LABELLE	F	19	Nko'olong	Bulu	Catholic	student	4 erne	Celibalaire	Arm fracture (left)	20/02/2022
30	EFFA MOISE	M	24	AKOK	BULU	EPC	Debrouillard	4th year	Celibalaire	Double Ira cl u re tibia perone (left)	28/01/2022
31	Francine	F	42	BIDOUIII	BULU	EPC	Menagere		Celibalaire	Ankle dislocation (right)	28/01/2022
32	CAROLE ANRIETTE	F	25	KRIBI EBWA	FANG	EPC	Menagere		celibalaire	Sick watch	19/11/2021
33		F	98							widow	Sick watch	19/11/2021

Appendix 5: Observation guide
I Presentation of the study context
The environment
Noise
The light
The workspace
The structure of the therapeutic village
Materials
The internal structure
Care items
Beds (materials)
Bed layout
The sick
II care activities
Welcoming patients (words, facial expressions, laughter, smiles).
Behaviour
The therapist
The patient
Sick guards
Gestures
The looks
Attention
1) Auscultation of the patient
1) The therapist's behaviour (gestures, facial expressions, speech, tone, etc.)
2) Patient behaviour (
Assessing the radio cliche
Behaviour,
Gestures,
Mimics
Words
Palpation of the body in pain
Gestures on the patient
Emotions and facial expressions
The lyrics
Making tools: the "Akang
The manufacturing material
Where it comes from
How it's made
How to use it
Preparation of the drug:
Types of medicines
Leaf typology (origin, quality
Type of bark (origin, quality, etc.)
Preparation items
Preparation
Preparing the leaves
Preparing the bark
Preparation of the powder
III the body at work
Traditional practitioner/patient interactions
Patient/patient interactions (speech, facial expressions, etc.),
Massages
The tools
Gestures
Traditional practitioner/patient interactions
The therapist's behaviour
Patient behaviour
Scarification

The gestures of the tradipratician
The tools
Emotions
The shape
Application of the drug
The gestures and expressions of screwing
Bandaging and immobilisation techniques
Positions and gestures
Rehabilitation
The process
The tools
Gestures
Objects
The shielding ritual
The process
What you need
The lyrics
Appendix 6: Film interview guide
Home
Can you tell me how your patients are received?
What items do you ask your patients for?
Why do you require your patients to have an X-ray?
Where do you get your knowledge of X-ray film analysis?
Consultation and diagnosis
What are the etiological circumstances of your patients?
Is there a mystical origin?
What is their perception of their state of health?
Preparing the medicine
How many elements are needed for the drug?
How long does a medicine take to prepare?
How does the medicine behave after application?
Massage and scarification
What massage techniques do you use during your treatment?
What tools do you use for massage?
Which positions for your patients?
What dangers do you run when using treatment tools such as razor blades? By frequently handling your patients' blood, do you have a clear feeling of being well protected? What are your means of protection?
Application of the drug and drying time
What role does this drug play in the body?
Why take so long to dry?
Bandaging and local immobilisation
Why immobilise a patient's fracture?
What impact does bandaging have on the fracture?
How long does local immobilisation last?
What role do the pieces of plywood and the 'Akang' play?
What other means of immobilisation are there?
Physical rehabilitation of joints
What are the stages in rehabilitation?
How long does rehabilitation last?
What equipment do you use for rehabilitation?
Who buys this equipment?
Shielding ritual
Why the shielding ritual?
What is the impact of this ceremony after a patient has been treated?
What is the symbolism of this ceremony? How effective is this ritual?
What are the advantages of shoring?
What are the disadvantages of shoring?
How can we ensure that this ceremony has an impact on the patient? How effective is this ritual?
What are the advantages of shoring?
What are the disadvantages of shoring?

Appendix 7: Interview guide for the two village traditional healers

Hello, my name is ZONGO MERIC and I'm a Master 2 research student in Visual Anthropology at the University of Ngaoundere. As part of the end of my Master's degree, I am currently carrying out a study on : The therapeutic village of ZE KANE Samuel: care practices for bone fractures in Niete. The aim of my work is to investigate and understand the reasons why patients suffering from bone diseases are referred to therapeutic villages, and at the same time to observe the practices used to treat these diseases in this therapeutic village. Shooting the film will enable us to showcase your expertise and see how you have integrated the knowledge of conventional medicine into your traditional care practices to make them more effective and efficient, with the aim of advocating that the positive aspects of bone fracture care, such as acupuncture, be incorporated into our heritage, or to see how the traditional therapist can work alongside the bone specialist or physiotherapist to reduce the cost of operations. I would like to talk to you about this and find out everything you know about it. Please be honest and sincere with me.

Investigator: ZONGO MERIC

Survey :

I. Life trajectory of the characters

Age

How old are you?

Where were you born?

Sex

Ethnic group

What ethnic group are you?

What languages do you speak? Or have you learnt these languages?

What is the name of your village?

School career

Have you studied

What is your level of education? Where have you studied?

Can you tell us about your educational background?

Why didn't you continue?

What did you do after your studies?

Social status

What use were these studies to you?

How long did you serve as... ?

Religion

What religion are you?

How did you become part of this religious community?

Is it a personal choice or the influence of those around you?

Why did you choose this confession

What is your perception of religion?

Do you practise traditional beliefs?

Does your religion prevent you from practising (traditional beliefs)?

Why do you use these two registers in your life?

What use is Western religion to you?

What about traditional religion?

Marital status

Are you married?

Tell me about your meeting

Under what regime?

Monogamy? Polygamy?

Why did you choose this regime?

Can you tell me the story of your manage, customary, religious or civil ceremony?

How old are you when you get married?

What is your wife's name?

Do you have any children?

How many children have you had?

How many boys?

How many girls?

What ages?

What about the spacing between the children?

What do they do?

Who among them is interested in the practice of care?

Who will inherit this therapeutic knowledge?

Family demographics

Who are your grandparents?
Who are your parents?
Do you have any brothers or sisters?
How many are still alive?
Who does your family live with?
Parents, grandparents, aunts, uncles, brothers, sisters, cousins
Who among them is interested in traditional medicine?

Spouse's occupation

What is your spouse's profession? Are you a friend?
Concubine?
Does he/she contribute to the costs?
How do we do it?

Means of transport

Do you have a means of locomotion? On foot? Motorbike? Car? How did you buy it? What does it do for you?

PRESENTATION OF THE ZE KANE THERAPEUTIC VILLAGE Samuel

How did you settle into the village?
Where did you get the idea to create this traditional hospital?
Can you tell me the story of this traditional hospital?
Did you have any problems setting up your business?
What are these difficulties?
Did you receive any help to set up your business?
Who was this help from?
What is your relationship with other traditional practitioners?
Are you an association? How do you operate?
Where did you get the idea of becoming a tradipratician (masseur)?
Tell me about the history of this profession
Is it a passion A gift?
Or did you learn it?
Where?
How did you learn?
Tell us about it? Where? How?
Have you paid for your training? If not, why not?
Why did you choose to become a traditional practitioner instead of doing something else?
How long have you been in the business?
Tell me about your first patients

ACTIVITIES IN CARE PRACTICE

How do you organise your working day?
What types of bone disease do you treat?
Sprains? Dislocations? Fractures?
How many patients do you see a day? Per month? Per year?
What is the age and sex of the patients?

Etiological circumstances of patients

In your opinion, what are the etiological circumstances of your patients?
What do your patients tell you?

Reason for consultation

Why do patients turn to traditional medicine?
Is it the difficult access to hospital?
Is it the low cost of traditional medicine that you're proposing?
Is it the belief in traditional medicine?
Or dissatisfaction with medical treatment?
What reasons do your patients give you?
Palpation of the suffering body

Types of bone disease

Can you tell me about the types of bone disease you know about?
Which ones are you looking after?

Types of lesions

What types of lesions do you treat?
Generally speaking, what are the sites of your patients' lesions?

Lesional auscultation of patients

How is a patient auscultated without an X-ray?
How do you auscultate a patient with an X-ray image?

Billing for the service
How much does it cost to treat a fracture?
How does it work? (by instalment or in full)
CARE PRACTICES PROPER
Manufacture of 1 bone repair tool
What tools do you have for patient care? How is the cage made?
What is its role?
Where does this material come from?
Preparing the medicine
What products are needed to prepare the medicine?
What types of remedies do you use?
Where does it come from?
Where do you get these products from?
How long does it take to prepare a medicine?
What is the result?
How are sprains treated?
Dislocations? Fractures? Where is the site of the lesion?
TREATMENT TIMES
What time do you treat fractures?
Why this time of day?
Is there a set time for receiving patients?
Why is this?
Do you treat all week?
If not, what days do you treat your patients?
What are the treatment stages for these diseases?
Are the treatments for these different illnesses different?
If not, why not?
How long does it take to treat a sprain or dislocation?
A fracture
What tools do you use?
What products do you use?
Auscultation of patients
How were consultations carried out in the beginning?
Do you rely on biomedicine when asking your patients for X-rays?
How did you introduce this modern medical practice?
How long have you been asking your patients for X-rays?
Have you studied radiology and medical imaging?
Explain to me how you come to interpret the images on the X-ray films
SCARIFICATION
What types of treatment do you offer your patients?
Is there a specific type of evil?
Why a razor blade for cuts?
Who buys razor blades?
How long does a razor blade last?
Why make the cuts on the patient's body every day?
Application of the drug
How long does it take to dry after applying the medicine? How effective is this medicine?
BANDAGE
Why do you bandage the lesion seat What are your bandaging techniques?
POSITIONING THE CLIP
What different patient immobilisation positions do you use?
How long can a patient be immobilised?
THE RISKS OF BEING A THERAPIST
Once you're in the thick of your work, what dangers are you exposed to? How do you deal with these obstacles?
Do these dangers have an impact on your body Your life?
Your entourage?
If yes, what impact do they have?
THE THERAPIST/PATIENT RELATIONSHIP
What is your relationship with your patients?
Are there any difficulties you encounter with your patients?
If so, which ones?

If not, why not?

Does the practice of treating bone diseases involve any prohibitions?

Which ones?

Why these prohibitions

What are the dangers for those who do not respect these prohibitions?

Do you have any prescriptions for your patients? Food?

Movements? Position?

If so, why?

PATIENTS' THERAPEUTIC ITINERARIES

How do you contact your patients?

Where do your patients come from?

What are your references?

What are the conditions for receiving patients?

Can you tell me where your patients come from?

What state are they in?

What are their reasons for doing so?

PATIENT MONITORING

How patients are monitored

LIMB REHABILITATION

How long will it take to rehabilitate your patients' joints?

How is this stage carried out?

Do you have the right equipment?

Where does this equipment come from?

ARMOURING RITUAL

What is the symbolism of the armouring ritual? What are the shielding tools? How is the shielding ritual performed? Why is the shielding ritual carried out after a patient has been treated?

Does sacrificing the chicken have an impact on the patient's life?

Difficult meetings

What difficulties have you encountered in the course of your work? How did you overcome these difficulties?

Employee satisfaction

How do you feel when you see a patient?

How do you feel after treating a patient?

Why do you feel this way?

Do you have the impression that your patients are grateful?

Why is this?

Appendix 8: Interview guide for patients

Hello, my name is ZONGO MERIC and I'm a Master 2 research student in Visual Anthropology at the University of Ngaoundere. As part of the end of my Master's degree, I am currently carrying out a study on : ZE KANE Samuel's therapeutic village: bone fracture care practices in Niete. The aim of my work is to investigate and understand the reasons why patients suffering from bone diseases are referred to traditherapeutes and, at the same time, to observe how these diseases are treated in this therapeutic village. I'd like to talk to you about this, to find out everything you experience and feel when you enter this therapeutic village. Please be honest and sincere with me.

Identification

Investigator's name: ZONGO MERIC

Name of survey :

1) . Age

How old are you?

2) . Sex

What gender are you?

3) . The ethnic group

What ethnic group are you from? Which ethnic group do you belong to? Fang? Beti? Bulu? If so, tell me about the history of your ethnic group? What makes your ethnic group special? What are the things that identify your ethnic group? Practices? Behaviour? Eating habits? Sexuality Clothing? Dances? Language ?

V - Marital status

Are you married, and if so, to whom? Tell me about your wedding ceremony, whether it was customary or religious. At what age?

If single, why? Do you want to?

Are you widowed? Divorced? Are you cohabiting? If yes, with whom? If not, why? Do you have a boyfriend or girlfriend? If so, do you want to get married?

Are you alone? If so, why?

VI The number of children in care

Do you have any children? If yes How many children do you have? How many girls/ Garmons?
What age? How far apart are the children?
If not, why not?

VII The number of people in charge of the house.
Father ? Mother ? Brother ? Other ? Why

VIII spouse's occupation
What is your spouse's profession? Friend? Concubine? Does he/she contribute to the expenses? If yes, how? If not, why?

IX Means of transport
Do you have a means of locomotion? On foot? Motorbike? Car? How did you buy it? What does it do for you?

XI Circumstances of the illness
Can you tell me under what circumstances you contracted this illness? Tell us about that day. Do you feel it was just an accident or something else? If anything else, please tell us.

THERAPEUTIC ITINERARY FOR PATIENTS
Where did you go after your accident? How long did you stay there? Why were you there? What were your reasons for changing facilities? Who brought you to Nko'olong? Why or why not?

XII ACCESS TO TRADITHERAPEUTE
What were your reasons for turning to traditional treatments? How did you get here? Who accompanied you? Why did you come? What ailment brought you here? Have you already received treatment from a traditherapeute? If not, why not? How do you find the reception and care? How do you rate the treatment time? Apart from traditional medicine, do you use any other medicine? If yes, why? What do you expect from your GP? Are there any difficulties accessing masseurs? If so, please explain. How do you rate the cost of treatment? Are you happy with it? If no, please explain
Please explain. Who will pay for your treatment? Have you kept all your appointments? If not, why not?

2- Reception conditions
Can you tell me how your therapist received you? How would you rate the welcome in this therapeutic village? Why or why not? What tools did the therapist ask you to use? Did you meet the therapist's requirements? Why or why not? How do you put yourself at ease? Do you have an assistant? Are you comfortable with the presence of other patients? How do you behave at the start?

3-Treatment/treatment relationship
How do you rate the treatment process? What are your expectations? What is your relationship with your therapist? Do you have any regrets about being in this traditional hospital? How do you feel during the massage? Are you afraid to use the blade every day? What technique do you use to reduce the pain you feel? How do you feel during the application of the medicine? Can you describe how you feel after the therapist has placed the barrette and bandaged the fracture?

PATIENT/PATIENT INTERACTIONS
Interactions: Are there ever conflicts in the common room? What can provoke conflict? How are conflicts resolved?

NUTRITION
How do you eat? How many times a day? Who feeds you? How do you organise your ration?

INSIDE THE DORMITORY
Business arrangements
Where do you keep your things? How do you find the space that welcomes you? Are you satisfied with the facilities available to you? Why or why not?
Who looks after your sleeping area?

Appendix 9: Interview guide for CMA healthcare staff
Hello, my name is ZONGO MERIC and I'm a Master 2 research student in Visual Anthropology at the University of Ngaoundere. As part of the end of my Master's degree, I am currently carrying out a study on : The therapeutic village of ZE KANE Samuel: bone fracture care practices in Niete. The aim of my work is to investigate and understand the reasons why patients suffering from bone diseases are referred to therapeutic villages, and at the same time to observe how these diseases are treated in this therapeutic village. The results of my research could help to improve the quality of care and management of patients suffering from bone diseases, both in hospitals and in therapeutic villages. I'd like to have a chat with you about this, to find out everything you experience and feel as soon as you enter this therapeutic village. Please be honest and sincere with me.

1) Identification
Name of interviewer: ZONGO MERIC
Name of the survey: what is your name?

2) Age
How old are you?

3) Gender
What gender are you?

4) The ethnic group
What ethnic group are you from? Which ethnic group do you belong to? Tell me about the history of your ethnic group? What makes your ethnic group special? What are the things that identify your ethnic group? Practices? Behaviour? Food? Sexuality? Clothing? Dances ? Rites? And rituals? Speech?

5) **School career**

What is your level of education? Primary? Secondary? University? Where did you study? Why didn't you go further with your studies?

6) **Religion**

What religion do you follow? Protestant? Catholic? tell me how you became one? What beliefs do you still hold dear? Why do you use these two religious registers?

7) **Marital status**

Are you married? Widowed, divorced? Single? If yes, married, widowed, divorced, single? At what age were you married? Widowed? Divorced? Single? Why single? With a woman of which ethnic group? Why or why not? Is it a customary marriage? Civil? Religious? Why customary? Civil, religious? And your beliefs? How many children do you have? How many daughters? How many gargons? Do they work? How many? What do the others do? How old is the first? How old is the last? Who are your parents? Are your parents still alive? If so, how many are still alive? If not, when did they pass away? What did they do ? How many brothers and sisters do you have ? How many are still alive? Do you have grandparents ? Aunts? Cousins? Cousins?

8) **Social status**

What job do you do? How long have you been doing it? Can you tell me about the history of your profession and how you got into it? Do you have any regrets about choosing this profession? Why or why not?

Spouse's occupation

What is your spouse's profession? Friend? Concubine? Does he/she contribute to the expenses? If yes, how? If not, why?

1) **Means of transport**

Do you have a means of locomotion? On foot? Motorbike? A car? What do you use it for?

2) **Presentation of the healthcare structure**

What is the name of your healthcare facility? Is it public, private or denominational? What category does your hospital fall into? What is the health map for your district? Can you tell me about it? How many staff does your hospital have? Which specialists do you have? Who deals with cases of bone disease? Why do you do this?

3) **Working with therapists**

Which organisations do you work with? For how many years? How is this collaboration going? Why do you want to work with us? What type of collaboration do you have? What is your perception of traditional healthcare structures? Do you have any cases referred by therapists? Do you have cases that you refer to traditional therapists? What are the different pathologies that you refer to traditional therapists? What are the reasons for this?

Types of fracture patients

Where do patients with physical trauma come from? Patients come from the place where the illness occurred - why do they come to you? Patients come from therapeutic villages Why do they come to you? Patients who go directly to you because they believe in modern medicine? What are the reasons?

V. Billing for patient care

How much does care cost? Do people pay by nature? What, for example? Do you ever treat patients for free because they are indigent? Why or why not? What is the treatment scale for fractures? Can you tell me about it? How many cases do you receive per day, week, month or year? What is the current number of fracture cases in your clinic?

Thank you for your clarification.

Appendix 10: Rights assignment contract

AUTHORISATION TO USE IMAGES AND SOUND

"Le village therapeutique de ZE KANE Samuel: pratiques des soins des maladies des os a Niete".

I, the undersigned, agree to be photographed for the

ethnographic research film mentioned in reference. I hereby give full permission to ZONGO MERIC Born 28/11/1994 in Adjap Matricule: 19B877LF student at the University of Ngaoundere Visual Anthropology. for the broadcasting, representation and all operations necessary for the academic and pedagogical exploitation of the audiovisual work on all or part of the recorded images and comments, for the production entitled "Le village therapeutique de ZE KANE Samuel: pratiques des soins des maladies des os a Niete", within the university framework, in the original/doubled or subtitled version, on any media and any support and by any process existing or unknown to date, without limitation of time, and free of charge. I guarantee Mr ZONGO MERIC against any recourse of any kind whatsoever.

My name may be mentioned in the credits of the audiovisual work, on the occasion of any educational or academic use of it.

Nko'olong le

Name and surname of speaker:

Date and place of birth :

Legal address :

Signature

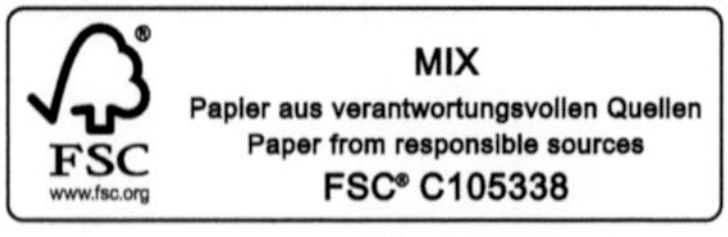

Printed by Books on Demand GmbH, Norderstedt / Germany